T0128194

SWEETER WITHOUT SUGAR

How to Break Free from the Sugar Habit
and Improve Your Quality of Life

JULIA YU

BALBOA.
PRESS
A DIVISION OF HAY HOUSE

Balboa Press books may be ordered through booksellers or by contacting:

Balboa Press
A Division of Hay House
1663 Liberty Drive
Bloomington, IN 47403
www.balboapress.com
1 (877) 407-4847

Print information available on the last page.

ISBN: 978-1-9822-3045-6 (sc)
ISBN: 978-1-9822-3046-3 (hc)
ISBN: 978-1-9822-3047-0 (e)

Library of Congress Control Number: 2019908746

Balboa Press rev. date: 06/28/2019

This book is dedicated to my dear husband, Kevin. I will never forget the day he told me I was sweeter without sugar and gave me the idea for the title of this book.

CONTENTS

Part 3: How to Make New Habits Stick

ACKNOWLEDGMENTS

A BIG THANK YOU goes to Traci Butz, my AMAZING Tony Robbins Results Coach, for helping me to break free from habits and patterns that have been holding me back for so many years. I would also like to send a BIG THANKS to all the Health Coach Institute success coaches who coached me while getting my health coach certification, especially Tracy Hjorth. The mental rehearsals we did together helped me build the self-compassion I needed to grow my heart. A special thanks to fellow health coaches Heidi Hochstetler for giving me great ideas on how to reimagine this book and Jennifer LaBonte for cheering me on every step of the way. Gratitude also goes to my parents, family, and friends, especially my husband, Kevin Yu, for his encouragement and support, as well as my sister, Silvia Suh, for showing me the path to wellness and helping me start my journey. Many thanks to the wonderful folks in the Office of Teacher Education, aka OTE Family, at Teachers College, Columbia University, for being excited for me as I ventured into the world of health and wellness. Huge thanks also go to the Balboa Press team for making my dream of helping people lead healthier and happier lives become a reality with the publication of this book.

A very special, loving thanks goes to my divine Grandmother. Her Korean name translates to the word *moon* in English, and whenever I saw the moon in the sky, I gathered the strength I needed to keep writing this book. She has taught me what it means to live with resilience, acceptance, and kindness.

INTRODUCTION

This book is intended to shed light on how our food habits impact our bodies and ultimately our quality of life. I always thought of myself as a mom with sugar issues, but when I realized that my quality of life was going downhill because of the food I was eating, I finally put in more effort and stopped taking the easy way out and giving into the cravings. I learned how to be *compassionate* with myself when cravings arose instead of *resist* them, and I have finally found peace with food, with myself, and with others. My life is wonderful now that I have broken free from my sugar habits, and it would make me so happy if your life becomes wonderful too after reading this book.

To all the other moms out there: It's time to slow down, step back, and ask ourselves what really matters in life. Life is sweeter when we can be more present in the moment.

To all the other closet eaters out there: It's time to come out and substitute fresh air and sunshine as food for the body, mind, and spirit. Reconnect with yourself and allow self-compassion to warm your heart.

To all the other yo-yo dieters out there: It's time to focus on healing your mind and stepping away from the guilt and shame. I have tried many different weight-loss programs and have finally learned that focusing on healing the mind and the heart allows weight loss to happen naturally. This is not a weight-loss book, but I was finally able to lose weight and keep it off after I got rid of the scale and started focusing on the healing process.

To all the other people out there with sugar habits: Life can be sweeter without sugar. You'll find out what this means once you commit to breaking free from your sugar habits.

It's never too late or too early to look at your life and prepare yourself for an even better way of living. Chronic pain and fatigue, pills, and unhappiness can all go away. It's time to break free from mental holds that have stopped you from living the life you want to live.

1
PART

HOW TO BECOME AWARE OF YOUR SUGAR HABITS

CHAPTER 1

How Can Breaking Free from the Sugar Habit Help?

For where there is awareness there is choice,
and where there is choice there is freedom.
—Mary O'Malley

Are you in the habit of looking for something sweet after dinner, after lunch, or all day long? Picture yourself eating or drinking that sweet something and hopping onto a roller coaster. The sugar stimulates your body, and your energy level goes up and hits a peak. All of a sudden, it drops down, and you crash. This keeps happening again and again, and you are left wondering when you get to go up again.

If the blood sugar roller coaster is not your thing, perhaps you'd like to ride the Ferris wheel or merry-go-round. You hop into the seat, and it takes you around and around in the same habit loop. You can't seem to get off, no matter how many times you try. It just keeps taking you around and around. You can't stop it because you are not the one in the control center—or are you, but you just don't know it yet?

Would you like to get off these rides and see what life can be like on a different kind of ride? This ride is built by you and is one you can call your own. On this ride, you can get on and off when you want to and be proud of building it.

In order to build a solid ride, you've got to build it one day at a time, one piece at a time. You must show up every day and own it. The ride is yours—only yours.

Then, when you are ready to share the ride with other people in your life, you get to have fun with them too.

What would make it strong so you don't fall off? In order to create a foolproof ride, you must develop a sense of awareness of how things work and how things are interconnected. You must set up the conditions for inevitable success.

Once awareness sets in, together with a greater understanding of why things do what they do, you can mindfully start putting the pieces together. After it's assembled, you may enjoy keeping things the same for a while, or you might want to expand it and transform it into something even more amazing.

Think possibilities. Think positivity.

If you can think about possibilities and think positively, you can build a ride that will last you a lifetime.

There will be moments when things get bumpy or scary, but you must think positively because your decisions will shape your actions. A positive mindset will lead to positive actions, and a negative mindset might cause you to take down the pieces unknowingly.

Are you ready to build your very own ride the way you want to? If the answer is yes, keep on reading and building. If your answer is maybe, perhaps something in the book will spark something in you to build a state-of-the-art ride after all. If your answer is no, please keep reading anyway, and perhaps you will stumble upon a nugget of gold that will give you the power to build something. What that something is will be up to you.

Why I Decided to Break My Sugar Habits

I was once in the habit of looking for a sweet something after dinner every day. I thought eating an orange rather than something full of sugar would be a better choice, but eventually, my disgruntled stomach told me that it wasn't such a great alternative after all. I felt like the orange was lodged in my stomach like a baseball on some nights and swirling around like a tornado on other nights. The fact that I was really bloated and looked like I was four months pregnant even though I wasn't didn't help either. But it was a habit to eat an orange, and it never occurred to me that eating it was making me feel ill.

Then on one random day, I came upon an article about a woman who quit sugar for three years and how this changed her life. Sarah Wilson became my inspiration, and her online program started me on my journey to living a life free of cravings, insatiable hunger, and pain. She made me realize that I was drawn to sugar through fruit, which was mind-blowing because everyone says that fruit is one of the best things to eat—but I realized that fruit was hurting my body. I would eat fruit in the morning for breakfast, midmorning, with and after lunch, and after dinner. I was constantly wondering what fruit or snack I would eat next, and food was the only thing on my mind all the time.

I accepted my body and the way it was before giving birth to two children. I gained fifty pounds with my first pregnancy and tried to lose as much of it as I could before the second pregnancy. But I wasn't able to go back to my original weight. I tried not to gain too much weight with my second pregnancy, but I ended up gaining another fifty pounds and was close to two hundred pounds by the time my son was born. I had never been that heavy, and I felt miserable carrying all the extra baggage. I tried all sorts of weight-loss programs, lost some weight, and gained some back. Eventually, the diet mentality and the I-deserve-a-sweet-treat mentality led to the overindulgence in junk food beyond belief. I kept telling myself that I would start over on Monday, but week after week passed, and I just kept feeling more and more defeated.

When I talked with other moms, wishing we could have our old bodies back always came up. But I learned that comparing my body to another mom's body did not help me in any way because it just made me feel worse about myself. So, I decided to stop comparing myself to other people, and I now feel much better about who I am.

After a long stretch of no sugar, I had some and then yelled at my kids for not cleaning up after themselves. After my rant, my daughter asked, "Mommy, did you eat sugar today?" I had to confess and apologized. I couldn't believe that my nine-year-old daughter recognized the symptoms of sugar in my system. Sugar causes mood swings, and I felt really bad about taking it out on her.

To all the other moms out there who have also felt bad about taking negative emotions out on their kids: breaking free from the sugar habit can ignite a new level of strength. Perhaps it can provide the energy to be more present with your kids; create new, fun family rituals and traditions; or set up a regular girls' night out if you are seeking connection on multiple levels. With this new level of depth, harmony, and satisfaction in all relationships, perhaps you can reinvent, restructure, or reimagine your career so you can create the lifestyle you truly desire or give back to your community in a more powerful way.

What I Noticed after Breaking Free from Sugar

After quitting sugar, my body deflated as if a balloon were slowly starting to lose air. My face thinned out, and my clothes felt looser. After the four-week mark, I noticed that the skin on my face was softer, and the dark circles under my eyes were disappearing. Even the wrinkles were fading! How could this be? My skin was glowing, and the aging process was reversing; this saved me money on expensive lotions and cleansers. Why buy stuff with carcinogens that will make my skin look worse down the road when I don't have to?

The pain in my knees and the achiness in my back vanished. I thought my back was achy because my mattress was old. If I had known that sugar was causing me back pain, I could have saved a lot of money and kept my mattress.

As I went into a deeper sleep on my new mattress, I slept through the night. (I also fell asleep more easily because sugar causes anxiety.) I woke up feeling as if I had the perfect amount of sleep and felt ready to conquer the world.

When I woke up with fresh energy, I noticed that my collarbones were showing and that I had shoulders. I'd thought they'd gone into hiding forever, but the continuous deflation was allowing them to show up again. It felt great to have more energy and add more movement into my life. I started doing exercises at home, and then I signed up for a sculpting class at a gym. Movement each week usually consisted of thirty to forty-five minutes of walking at least five days a week and one hour of sculpting a week. The benefits of walking are tremendous, and I could write a whole book on that too.

The removal of processed food and increase in movement led to the disappearance of cellulite from my thighs. Who would have thought this could be possible? My belly area deflated, and the appearance of my waist and weight loss happened naturally without the stress of having to try. Life was absolutely fabulous.

Tight, achy shoulders stopped being a problem and so did what I thought were arthritic hands. I thought that years of playing the flute and typing too much were catching up to me in my forties, but that wasn't the case at all. The chronic pain I had been feeling for years started to fade and is completely gone now.

I no longer had cracking and bleeding hands because of the cold temperatures in the winter; this was also a big plus. Sugar causes a lot of skin problems in general, including eczema and acne.

On top of all the wonderful physical effects, my mental clarity was incredible. I took a summer intensive course that required three hundred pages of reading in one week, and I actually read every page and understood the material. When I was in college, I read the same paragraph five times and still couldn't remember what I had read. If I could go back in time and know what I know now about the impact of refined food on the mind, I would have been much more mindful and tried to make better choices with food. It was as if I had become Julia version 2.0 without the constant pressure behind my eyes and the dull headaches from looking at the screen for long periods of time.

But what I loved most of all was the freedom.

Freedom from the obsession with food and the insatiable hunger allowed me to focus on improving other aspects of my life.

What would you like freedom from? If you want to break free from pills, your couch, your unhappy state of mind, or something else that is stopping you from living the life you desire, here's your chance to break free from habits that don't serve you and start building habits that will improve your quality of life.

The new energy I felt also propelled me to initiate more projects at work and lead them. I also spoke up more at meetings, and I felt like I could contribute in different ways at work where I didn't before.

Who was this new person? She was someone who finally broke free from the sugar habit and created newer, better habits.

By discovering nourishing foods that provide the most energy for your body and turning healthy habits into behaviors that last, your mind and your body can experience a whole new level of strength, energy, and vitality. This new kind of energy can actualize the lifestyle you have always wanted, which can include experiencing peak health, peaceful relationships, a stable financial foundation, and a fulfilling career. Otherwise, feeling drained and disconnected from yourself and everyone around you could become the norm if it isn't already. I invite you, dear reader, to see how your effort and investment in your health can impact every area of your life regardless of your age, hair color, or astrological sign.

One way to improve our quality of life is by improving the way we talk to ourselves. Positive self-talk can lift our spirits, make us believe that we are capable, and *allow* us to be at peace with ourselves. On the other hand, negative self-talk can be destructive and *stop* us from being at peace with ourselves.

I started to text myself and the universe encouraging words such as, "I can do this," in order to stay positive.

Some people use the word *universe* as a synonym for a higher being, but in this book, when I refer to the universe, I am simply referring to a vast open space where anything could happen at any time. Sending positive vibes to the universe will lead to favorable outcomes if you believe it will.

I invite you to do the same by texting yourself the answer to the question posed at the end of each chapter to keep you focused and positive when you build your ride. Add yourself as a contact on your phone and create an amusing nickname for yourself to keep it lighthearted.

Please stick to only using positive statements in your texts. If you are feeling down and negative, allow yourself to feel the emotion and pose a question to yourself such as, "Why am I feeling this way?" rather than, "What's wrong with me?" Start to build your awareness by asking questions and being curious.

Send a text message to the universe by answering this question: How would breaking free from the sugar habit help me?

CHAPTER 2

Why Do We Do What We Do? Is What We Do Helping Us or Hurting Us?

*Self-awareness doesn't stop you from making mistakes;
it allows you to learn from them.*

Almost half of our behaviors are automatic and are done repeatedly without much thought on any given day. I know of someone who wakes up and eats yogurt for breakfast every single morning. Starting the morning eating sugar and dairy can wreak havoc on the body, but many people aren't aware of this. Feeling tired and not having energy is what it is. Sugar and dairy also cause migraines, sinus problems, and anxiety. So if you are sitting in a meeting and can't focus on what the person is saying because of a headache or anxiousness, you've got to wonder why. What if it doesn't have to be this way?

We have been programmed to think that certain foods are good for us, especially dairy because it contains calcium. But did you know that many yogurts have a lot of *added* sugar and that sugar could cause breast cancer? Did you also know that the United States has the highest rate of osteoporosis because of the overconsumption of dairy? The ads showing friendly looking cows and slogans like "Milk: It Does the Body Good" have made us fall for the idea that dairy products are good for the body, but are they really? When people go on elimination diets to figure out the cause of their woes, there's a reason why dairy is always one of the first on the list to eliminate. Milk was meant to be had by calves, not humans, and that's why we can't digest it properly and should stay clear from it. If we don't buy it, the companies won't make it. Doing this can also prevent the torture and inhumane treatment cows have to undergo in order to produce milk.

The good news is that companies are producing more alternatives to dairy, such as almond milk, coconut milk, and hemp milk. I had to try five different brands of cheese before I found some I could actually swallow, but now I am happy to have found an alternative to dairy so the cows can be protected. We always have choices, even when we don't think we do.

Why Do We Do What We Do?

The brain's job is to keep us safe and protected. Any new activities could be dangerous and must be done cautiously or not at all. In order to overcome this hesitation and resistance, we must keep telling our bodies that we feel safe with the new activity. So if we usually start the day with a sugary cereal and milk and want to switch to a Dr. Praeger's spinach cake, chances are that the brain will tell us that the cereal and milk are the way to go. Even though we know better as we educate ourselves more, knowledge does not lead to behavior change. However, if we think of knowledge as potential power, we will know what we need to do to *ignite* the behavior change.

Knowledge does not equal behavior change.

Knowledge equals potential power to ignite behavior change.

In order for behavior change to occur, the brain needs reassurance that it is okay to change things up. This reassurance can happen in the form of praise and a little celebration with every little accomplishment. If part of your new routine is to drink a cup of warm water instead of juice in the morning, then it's important to celebrate this by acknowledging that you did it and letting the serotonin get into the brain. This may seem silly, but overlooking this will prevent the new habit from becoming ingrained in the brain.

The brain has a lot of different ways to keep us safe. Some of those methods are through automatic behaviors, which show up as habits that help us lead our everyday lives, and other behaviors can come out as compulsions, addictions, or urges to behave in a certain way even though they go against our better judgment and conscious wishes. We all have needs, and in order to meet those needs, we sometimes behave in ways that are inexplicable. But what if there is an explanation?

Six Human Needs

Anthony (Tony) Robbins, a motivational speaker and author, mentions that all human beings have six needs that must be met in his audio program *Unleash the Power Within.* They are the need for 1) certainty, 2) uncertainty, 3) significance, 4) connection, 5) growth, and 6) contribution.

The first four needs are *basic* in that we need to have *certainty* about having things such as a bed to sleep on every night. This sense of certainty provides us with a feeling of safety. On the other side of certainty, is *uncertainty*, or variety. Knowing that there will be food at home allows us to feel safe, but eating the same thing day after day can lead to a lack of variety, and most of us need variety in our lives in order to keep things interesting. The third need is *significance*, which refers to the need to feel like we matter and that we are important. Some people do this by trying to accumulate large amounts of money. They associate being rich with being significant. The fourth basic need is *connection*, or love. We need to feel like we belong and that someone cares for us (that someone could even be you through self-love).

In order to live a *fulfilling* life, not just an ordinary one, we need to meet the last two needs, which are growth and contribution. *Growth* can be sought through various resources and methods that allow us to stretch and build on what we already know and can do. The last one is *contribution* beyond self and to others. Millionaires could have all the luxuries in the world but not feel fulfilled because they either feel that they have stopped growing or because they feel that what they are doing is not helping others in a meaningful way. There is a lot more that goes into understanding the human psyche and how these needs play into our behaviors. Anthony Robbins has written multiple books such as *Awaken the Giant Within* and audio programs such as *Unleash the Power Within* that explain these concepts in greater depth.

In order to fully understand why we do what we do, we need to understand what the most important needs in our lives are, what our beliefs are, and the emotions that we habitually become addicted to according to the *Creating Lasting Change* audio program by Tony Robbins. Different people will put certain needs at the top of their priority lists, and that is what drives their behavior. Essentially, our beliefs drive our decisions, and our decisions drive our actions.

This book will hopefully spark an aha moment or new insight that will lead to a greater understanding of how the brain and body are interconnected. Thus, Brain Activation Mode (BAM) moments have been placed throughout the book to allow for some pausing and reflecting in order to build your state-of-the-art ride. Responses to BAM moments can be placed on a separate sheet of paper, journal, phone, or just in your head. I would strongly recommend writing them down to activate different parts of your brain as you think through the questions, but the choice is yours as the reader and thinker.

= Brain Activation Mode = BAM

Take a moment to review the list of the six human needs. If possible, write all six of them down on your own sheet. They are: 1) certainty, 2) uncertainty, 3) significance, 4) connection, 5) growth, and 6) contribution. Now circle the top two needs that you feel are most important to you in your life right now. In your eyes, what is life about?

If you would like to dig deeper into your brain, there will be opportunities to go beyond BAM and answer more complex questions. I will leave it up to you to decide whether you would like to build your ride starting from the ground up, which would entail answering BAM questions, or to go beneath the surface and make your way up, which would entail answering BAM and Beyond BAM questions.

Think possibilities.

= Beyond BAM =

If possible, give an example of how the two needs you selected as priorities play out in your life through your thoughts, beliefs, or actions.

In order to create lasting change, ask yourself these questions:

- What do I need?
- What do I want?
- What's getting in the way of what I want? (This could be physical barriers or mental ones, such as your beliefs or state of mind.)
- How is this solvable?

The answers to these questions are what drives your behaviors and your habits.

Paying Attention to Our Bodies' Signals

Does the dessert after dinner fill your need for *certainty*? Does your brain tell you that you have worked hard and deserve a reward? This is simplifying things tremendously, but perhaps things that you do have more meaning than you originally thought.

A habit-tracking chart will be provided later in the book to track your sugar habits. Once you track them and look for patterns, you will be invited to decide how you would like to meet your top needs.

One of the easiest ways to know if you need to outgrow a habit is if it causes pain or discomfort. For example, if your stomach starts to swirl every time you eat an orange after dinner like mine did, then it's a habit that needs some shifting (unless you want to feel uncomfortable every night). According to the principles of Ayurveda, fruit ferments or rots in your stomach as it is being digested, so I decided to replace the sweet fruit with something salty to try to break free from sugar. I needed an alternative, and at that point in time, that was the only thing in the pantry. I should have spent more time looking for a better alternative because as I reflect back, replacing sweetness with saltiness led to its own set of problems. Later on, salty foods were what I sought out constantly, and it took a while to break free from that too.

If you are not familiar with Ayurveda, it is the ancient study of a holistic or whole-body approach to healing through the study of how food impacts the body.

When I learned that fruit should be eaten separately from a meal because of the fermentation process, I decided to cut down on my fruit intake and started feeling better. Although the benefits of eating fruit include the additional vitamins and nutrients, the overconsumption of it could have a negative impact on the body because of the high fructose content in some fruits, and for me, it also acted as an appetite stimulant. This book is not intended for you to stop eating a particular food; instead, it is intended for you to learn how food impacts *your* body. If something makes you feel ill, it may be best to eat it in smaller portions, differently from the way it was eaten before, or not at all.

Is What We Do Helping Us or Hurting Us?

When we are mad, sad, glad, bored, or emotional, we have a tendency to head toward food for comfort. It takes away the pain, fills that void, and won't judge us. Another common habit is to start the day with caffeine, and it usually includes something sweet in the form of sugar, honey, or things like agave (which is considered by some people to be as bad or worse than sugar because it is more than 70 percent fructose). In the short run, going to sugar to pick us up does the job, but in the long run, could it be hurting us to be doing this?

I will be referencing habits in terms of being *helpful* or *hurtful* rather than *good* or *bad*. I will also be referencing food as *sugary* or *fresh* rather than *good* or *bad*. Categorizing food or people as being *good* or *bad* is not a healthy mindset because it infers judgment.

Energy Scale

On a scale of 1 to 10, do you have enough energy to get everything you need to get done? (A score of 10 equals a big *yes*.)

If you chose an 8, 9, or 10, you are thriving and should be very proud of yourself!

If you chose a 7, 6, or 5, you are struggling and could use more energy.

If you chose a 4, 3, 2, or 1, you are dragging along, and your quality of life could be suffering.

If you answered zero or a negative number, something has got to change. But people who need the most help in developing healthier habits are the *most resistant* to change, so it's important to start with a teeny, tiny step that is easy and doable.

This book will try to get you to where you can thrive beyond the score of 10!

Mr. Grouchy

My husband used to put six packs of sugar in his coffee every morning; otherwise, he became Mr. Grouchy. He claimed that his migraine wouldn't allow him to get things done around the house on the weekends if he didn't drink his coffee first. When I told him his addiction to caffeine and sugar was not helping him, a spark must have gone off in his brain because he went from six packets to five packets to four to zero. Then he realized the coffee creamer had sugar, so he left that out too. Then he realized he didn't like drinking coffee black, so he cut down to half a cup and transitioned to green tea and then to herbal tea. This blew me away because he is such a creature of habit (and a computer science person who needs logical steps). His habits are so ingrained that the thought of changing something would lead to revolts and fights between us. I just planted a little seed in his head, and he decided to do it on his own, in his own terms, and at his own pace.

Making a change too fast and without full buy-in from the brain can lead to feelings of loss of enjoyment and deprivation, and then tweaking a habit will become a temporary thing instead of something that evolves over time. Let's not scare the brain too much with too many changes too fast. If it doesn't feel safe, it will start to resist and tell you that you cannot live if you don't have sugar (which is not true). You will survive, and you will thrive!

Beliefs and Myths Ingrained in American Culture because of Mass Marketing and the Media

The major food companies that make huge profits do a ton of research on what makes food appealing to the masses through the careful study of texture, smell, and visual appeal. It's incredible how every little piece of that thing you ate has been carefully designed so you will want more of it. This way, companies guarantee themselves loyal customers for life.

The constant commercials showing sugary foods are designed to entice everybody to go down the junk-food aisle. A lot of kids begin their days with sugary cereals that have five to ten different kinds of sugars and artificial coloring. Products like these will eventually impact brain function negatively. Then we expect them to focus and sit still for hours at school. They will probably fill up on juice or something sweet again during lunch or snack time, and then at night after dinner, dessert will stimulate their system yet again. So they constantly wake up tired from all the crashes.

When I became aware of the impact of sugar on the body, I stopped buying juice boxes, soda, and cook___s. (The names of sugary items will not be typed out in most cases in order to be sensitive to readers who are triggered by these types of words like I am.) Believe it or not, the kids did not complain. They asked why they didn't see it in the house anymore, and I explained that I wanted them to be able to focus at school.

My son came home one day and told me that he was able to focus more in his classes, which made my day. Other moms who have experimented with the reduction of sugar have noticed that their kids get sick less and don't end up missing as many days of school. Sugar weakens the immune system. I would recommend doing a little experiment and seeing the results for yourself.

In the 1980s, commercials by a medicine company said that, "You've got to feed a cold." I totally believed this, and whenever I got sick, I would eat as much as possible even if I didn't want to. Now that I am older and a little wiser, I have learned that the last thing we should do is eat when we are sick because the blood goes to the digestive system to break down the food instead of going to the place that needs attention and healing. Sleeping is the best way to heal because the body heals when we are in a state of rest.

Another marketing technique that has ingrained itself in American culture is the concept that dinner is not complete without a sweet ending. My daughter used to say that half of her stomach was for dinner and half of her stomach was for dessert. We used to laugh about this, but now our habits have changed when we go out. We always drink water, and we only order dessert for a special occasion. Saving room for dessert is no longer a must.

American culture makes us think that we are being cheap if we don't order a sugary beverage at a restaurant. Companies make billions of dollars in profits from the sweet syrup in carbonated liquid. Their advertisements have been persuasive and powerful, but what if we told them that we choose to make our health a priority and don't buy it?

All the drinks and desserts from different outings and all the crashes from the blood sugar roller coaster rides will take its toll. It can take years to develop diabetes or cancer or chronic pain, so the key is to be preventive. Less than 10 percent of cancers are genetic. Adults eat in the same way as they did as children, so if a soda was at every meal in childhood, there's a pretty good chance that soda will be present in adulthood.

We live in a society that is obsessed with numbers and how things look.

What if we put our energy and attention into how we feel and think instead?

The media says we have to *fix* ourselves before we can be *outstanding*. But what if we no longer believed this, and we *stand out* in our own way according to our own personal standards?

Text message to the universe: What can I do to prevent the media from influencing my thoughts?

CHAPTER 3

What's the Deal with Sugar and Artificial Sweeteners?

We've been hoodwinked about sugar. We've had companies who rely on sugar like the big soda companies paying scientists to say that saturated fat was making us unhealthy causing heart disease and obesity, and not actual sugar. And so our eye has been off the ball for many, many years having a different villain, but really the villain has been sugar.

—Vani Hari

What counts as sugar? Every person you ask will give a different answer. Some people only see the white powdered stuff as sugar or sucrose. Others will say that anything that is high in fructose counts too. Anything that ends in *-ose* is a type of sugar, and if you see anything on the ingredient list that ends with *-ose* or any of the other names in this chapter, proceed with caution and try to opt for something without it. Dr. Susan Peirce Thompson, founder of Bright Line Eating, says that if sugar is not one of the first three ingredients, it does not cause the same type of dopamine response in the brain, so it is all right to eat that food. But you should listen to your body. Even if sugar is fifth on the list, if it still causes cravings, it's something you should probably avoid. There are so many choices when it comes to food. Choose something that comes from the earth that will nourish your body versus something from a factory. Your body will thank you.

There are a lot of hidden sugars in foods like cold cuts, pasta sauces, and canned soups. As I mentioned earlier, a large amount of sugar also hides in yogurt. If you look at the ingredient list, you'll see different types of sugar listed in addition to lactose. Did you know that more than half of the people in the United States and the world at large are lactose intolerant, and a huge percentage of those people don't even know it? The food you put in your body plays a *huge* role in how you feel physically and mentally.

The thing about sugar is that sometimes you can feel the effects of it pretty quickly. But you can't exactly feel your immune system weakening (unless you get sick often, which is a big sign) or that your brain is degenerating (unless you feel forgetful and absentminded a lot even though you are only in your twenties or thirties). If that's the case, lack of sleep or stress could be factors, but the food you are eating is probably a big factor.

Food companies and the media encouraged us to eat a low-fat diet starting in the 1970s and that has stuck until now. But it's time to make that unstick. Foods that are low in fat contain a lot of added sugars. Then there was the trans-fat scandal in packaged food, and companies came out with baked chips. The ingredient list on baked chips is actually worse than real potato chips. People have been gaining weight because of the so-called healthier version of certain foods. If we look at the ingredients, it's not healthier. It's just not.

The lack of fat consumption is also another cause for brain degeneration. The brain needs fat for continued growth. There are healthy fats from avocados and coconut oil, and there are the unhealthy ones from meat and deep-fried foods. Saturated fat from meat, chicken, dairy, and other animal products produces a set of similar illnesses as sugar, such as heart disease and cancer.

When I stopped buying sugary stuff, the cost of groceries decreased tremendously, which was a big plus. Buying a can of chickpeas and making my own roasted chickpeas by tossing them with some oil and salt and putting them in the toaster oven for about thirty minutes is so much cheaper than a bag of chips. Eating only three meals a day and not snacking really helps to cut down on grocery costs too. Not having to figure out what to snack on between meals has taken away a big chunk of my stress. According to Ayurveda, eating only three meals a day is best so that the digestive system has a chance to rest and take a break from all the work required in breaking down the food.

Different Names for Sugar

There are about sixty different names for sugar. Some of them are below:

Agave nectar, barley malt, beet sugar, brown sugar, cane juice, caramel, coconut sugar, corn sweetener, date sugar, dextrin, dextrose, fructose, fruit juice, glucose, high-fructose corn syrup (HFCS), honey, malt syrup, maltodextrin, maltose, maple syrup, molasses, palm sugar, rice syrup, saccharose, and, last but not least, sucrose (the carcinogenic white powdered stuff with no nutritional value).

Note: Anything on a nutrition label that has the word *syrup* next to it is up to no good, in addition to anything that ends with the letters *-ose*.

Artificial Sweeteners

If sugar is not the way to go, what about artificial sweeteners? They are actually worse and can cause even more damage to your brain and body. If you are in the habit of drinking a diet soda as a meal or drinking it with a meal, ask yourself if this habit is helping you or hurting you. Drinking a soda does not count as a meal. It can fill you up, and it's cheap, but our bodies naturally look for a meal. So if you don't eat lunch and drink a soda instead, your brain is going to wonder when and where that meal is, and it won't rest until it finds it. Diet sodas are actually worse because they can be more than three hundred times sweeter than sugar, which sends the brain into overload. Below is a list of reactions people have to aspartame, which is one of the more common artificial sweeteners found in diet sodas and gum.

Aspartame can cause minor and major life-threatening conditions that include:

- Abdominal and joint pain
- Cancer
- Damage to brain cells
- Depression
- Formaldehyde buildup
- Heart issues
- Infertility
- Insomnia and sleep problems
- Memory loss
- Vision problems

Sugar and artificial sweeteners have both been proven to be carcinogens. They are poisonous in their own ways. Even though it could cause cancer, sugar is still abundant, cheap, and easily accessible. Sugar has been compared to other harmful substances such as cigarettes. Decades ago, there were rumblings that smoking was not good for your health, but it wasn't a big deal until the number of people with lung cancer started to rise and awareness was instilled in people. It's the same with sugar now. There are rumblings, but most people are choosing to ignore them. But as more studies and stories show up in the news about the damage sugar is causing to society, there will be an uproar. If you are not the type to roar, you can avoid purchasing sugary foods. This in and of itself sends a message.

> **When people in a society have difficulty creating offspring because of artificial sweeteners that come in innocent-looking pink, yellow, and blue packages, there's a *huge* problem at the societal level.**

There needs to be more awareness about the impact of harmful substances that cause infertility and birth defects.

Artificial Sweeteners in Household Products

Almost all brands of toothpaste, mouthwash, and kids' vitamins have artificial sweeteners, so it is very important to look at the ingredient lists on these types of products. I couldn't believe it when I saw sweeteners in shampoos and lotions as well. Anything that touches the skin enters the bloodstream within thirty seconds, so it is best to avoid products with sweeteners.

Names of Artificial Sweeteners

Words that end in *-tol* are usually a type of artificial sweetener, but other words such as *saccharin* and *acesulfame potassium* are also sweeteners, so please be aware of what you are putting *in* and *on* your body.

High-Fructose Corn Syrup

High-fructose corn syrup (HFCS), otherwise known as corn sugar, is the chemically manipulated version of corn and can be found in bread, juices, pizza sauce, and many other foods. HFCS is also something to be on alert for and dodge because it can cause liver damage and many other types of problems. According to *The Blood Sugar Solution* written by Dr. Mark Hyman, high doses of fructose punch holes in the intestinal lining, allowing toxic gut bacteria to enter the bloodstream.

High-Sugar Foods

The recommended sugar intake for children is 3–6 teaspoons; for women, 6 teaspoons; and for men, 9 teaspoons. In order to see how many teaspoons of sugar is in something, divide the number of grams of sugar by 4. For example, some low-fat yogurts can have up to 48 grams of sugar. So you would divide 48 by 4 and get 12 teaspoons of sugar.

So the one yogurt is more than enough for the day, but many people don't stop there. The average person eats 22 teaspoons a day!

Guess how many teaspoons of sugar are in soda. One can of soda typically has 10–12 teaspoons of sugar. It is said that 90 percent of children drink at least one soda a day, which is astounding, and one in two adults drink at least one soda every day. Soda has been known to cause loss of bone mineral density because of the phosphoric acid, which is yet another reason to stay away from it.

How about swapping sodas, energy drinks, juices, and sweetened teas for noncaffeinated herbal teas or, dare I say it, *water*? I used to stay away from tea because I thought Lipton was the only kind of tea that existed until I went to the supermarket and looked at the tea aisle. It is one of my favorite places to browse. They have so many different flavors and aromas. If you prefer to drink tea cold, simply put the tea bag in cold water instead of hot water. Easy!

Other foods with added sugars include granola, orange juice, mayonnaise, and ketchup. Protein bars and sports drinks are extremely high in sugar. If you work out for three hours a day and wonder why you are not becoming leaner, the sugar is probably making you hold onto the visceral fat.

Sugary items will raise your blood sugar levels and put you back on the roller coaster. Other refined products like flour will do the same thing but faster, actually. A lot of people are getting away from wheat flour because of the gluten, which is indeed toxic, but they are heading toward gluten-free products, which typically have rice flour, potato starch, corn starch, or tapioca starch at the top of the ingredient list. These items actually spike blood sugar levels faster than sugar and wheat flour according to Dr. William Davis, author of *Wheat Belly*. I used the *Wheat Belly Journal* to track my wheat intake and study the impact it had on my body, and I must say, it was really, really helpful. I have put it on the list of recommended readings at the back of this book.

Educating Kids

I believe our job as parents is to educate our kids. One way to do this is by watching YouTube videos on the effects of sugar or a documentary as a family. The kids will resist, but there are a lot of short videos on the internet and great documentaries like *Carb-Loaded* on Food Matters TV (fmtv.com). My kids resisted, but then they actually enjoyed it and learned something from it.

The number of junk food ads kids watch every year is an astounding six thousand, so teaching them that the media is powerful and that we shouldn't believe everything they say is important in order to start turning them into savvy consumers.

By not allowing the obsession with sugar to grow as they get older, we can prevent twenty-year-olds from having heart surgery. Sugary beverages are the biggest source of sugar, so not bringing them into the house can make a big difference. If you can pass on buying the soda and juice, you will be doing everyone a big favor.

Sugar and Babies

Infant formula has sugar, and a mother's breast milk will very likely have sugar as well. If a liking to sweetness begins in infancy, there is a very high chance this inkling will continue for many years and decades. This generation of babies is expected to have shorter lives than their parents because of the food and lifestyle choices they will make as children and later as adults. The abundance of processed, cheap foods combined with a sedentary lifestyle because of phones and laptops will have tragic consequences if children do not develop healthy habits early in life. Teaching kids to become aware of how food impacts their bodies is something they can take with them through life.

Millennials are said to be the most depressed and anxious out of all the generations so far, which is also a result of food and lifestyle choices. Sugar and other refined foods cause our minds and bodies to become addicted to things in ways that seem pleasing but, in reality, are making people sick, depressed, and obese.

As more children and adults develop diabetes and other autoimmune diseases as a result of inflammation and weakened immune systems because of the food choices, we need to bring more awareness to this epidemic.

Ninety percent of diseases are caused by food, stress, and other environmental factors. It doesn't have to be this way if we bring more mindfulness and awareness to how things impact our bodies. Type 2 diabetes can be reversed in thirty days. Cancer can disappear without chemotherapy. This can all happen if people make better choices in food according to Dr. Mark Hyman in his book *The Blood Sugar Solution*.

Why Swap Food?

Researchers are saying that too much added sugar can lead to constant high blood sugar levels and put people at an increased risk of kidney disease.

A high intake of fructose can lead to obesity, which will make the heart work harder, as well as lead to high blood pressure, high blood fats, type 2 diabetes, and arterial dysfunction. These syndromes could also lead to an increased risk in developing dementia.

It's time to get off the roller coaster; stop the mood swings, cravings, and energy crashes; and start looking for nourishing foods.

Be careful with swapping sugar for protein or fat in meat. According to the book *Diet for a New America* by John Robbins, proteins and fats from meat lead to their own share of health risks, such as cancer and heart disease. There is a 0 percent death rate of people who died from lack of protein in developed countries like the United States. The best athletes in the country eat plant-based diets and do not eat meat. It is time to dispel myths that people who do not eat meat are weaklings because, in actuality, their endurance and performance are quite remarkable.

Below are some suggestions for food swaps:

- Choose olive oil infused with herbs over store-bought salad dressing.
- Choose nut butters over peanut butter or other sweet spreads.
- Choose almonds over crackers.
- Choose zoodles (zucchini noodles) over pasta.
- Choose a Dr. Praeger's veggie burger over a hamburger.

> It all comes down to making the better choice.
> Listen to what your body is telling you
> after you eat the food you chose.

Text message to the universe: When can you make time to look for a new, healthier option of a food to try?

Note about cell phones: If you have been sending text messages to the universe with your cell phone in your bedroom, please don't get into the habit of leaving the cell phone near your head while you sleep. Wireless waves from your cell phone are very harmful, and we don't want to add more toxins to the body.

CHAPTER 4

How Do I Become Aware of My Habits?

*You must learn a NEW WAY to THINK before
you can master a new way to BE.*
—Marianne Williamson

When you wake up in the morning, what is the first thing that you do? Is it to press the snooze button over and over again? Why do you do this? Is it because you feel too tired to get up?

Pressing the snooze button was what I used to do until I decided that it was a waste of time, and I might as well use the extra time sleeping instead of being irritated by the beeping noise.

But then I found a way to feel as if I had the perfect amount of sleep and wake up as if I could conquer the world. This is the truth! How did I finally reach this point? It happened after breaking free from the sugar habit and no longer waking up with the aftereffects of a sugar crash.

Contrary to what people believe, a new habit is not formed in twenty-one days. It can take up to 250 days to create new, long-lasting habits. Some say the average is sixty-six days.

The number of days it takes to create a new habit differs by person and how important it is to that person to change the behavior.

By learning to observe and become aware of the cues and rewards surrounding a habit, we can change the routines, according to Charles Duhigg, author of the book *The Power of Habit*. A typical habit loop consists of a cue (smelling coffee), routine (pouring a cup), and then a reward (drinking it). Sometimes the reward itself is not what drives us; it is the *anticipation* of the reward.

The key to habit change is building awareness around the cues and the rewards, recognizing the routine, and then figuring out whether this is a positive or negative way to meet a certain need. If it is a negative way to meet the need, figuring out an empowering alternative to meet that same need can lead to the golden ticket. Drinking coffee activates the dopamine response in the brain, which causes cravings and makes people search for a reward. If the reward you are seeking is relief from the stresses of life, could that relief come in a different form? If yes, what could that form be, and what could be a new routine to get to that reward? These are all questions we will continue to explore throughout the book.

You can't change what you don't acknowledge.

In order to transform our habits, we need to be aware of what they look like. You may be drinking six diet sodas a day and not even realize it! One serving is 8 ounces (oz), or one cup, and a standard can is more than 8 ounces.

Why Is Building Self-Awareness Important?

If we are aware of what we are *feeling* and *being* and *doing* as it happens, it can help us learn more about ourselves and our patterns, which will lead to an increase in self-awareness, self-regulation, and self-control. Becoming aware of the pattern sparks the pattern-breaking process.

In this book, self-awareness refers to the ability to connect our inner thoughts and feelings to external factors and understand how they impact our minds and our bodies. Self-regulation refers to our ability to manage our behaviors, emotions, and thoughts without outside assistance. An example of self-regulation would be limiting how much we eat on our own accord. The definition of self-control in this book is very similar to self-regulation in that it refers to our ability to manage our behaviors, especially when it comes to impulses and refraining from acting on them. Poor self-regulation has been seen as the cause for millions of American adults to continue to smoke and for more than half of the population in this country to qualify as overweight or obese.

> It's really important to understand the interconnectedness of the gut, mind, and body in order to be able to increase self-awareness and improve self-regulation.

Serotonin is known as the chemical in the brain that makes us feel happy. In recent years, scientists have found that gut bacteria help to produce serotonin, and it can be found in the lining of the stomach and intestines. So what we eat affects the production of serotonin, and low levels of serotonin have been linked to depression and other mood disorders, while high levels of serotonin have been linked to osteoporosis.

According to Kelly McGonigal's book *The Willpower Instinct*, the average person makes around two hundred food choices a day. When we make choices from a stance rooted in self-awareness, it allows us to take on a nonjudgmental approach rather than a critical one.

Honoring Hunger and Fullness

While I was getting my health coach certification through the Health Coach Institute, I learned about honoring hunger and fullness. When our bodies start to give us signs that we need food, such as a little gurgling noise, it's important to honor that sign. Start thinking about what to eat and where to get food when the hunger scale is around a 2 or 3 out of a scale of 10. Try to seek out a meal that will provide nourishment and positive energy, and eat at a 5 or 6 on the scale. If we wait until our hunger is a 10 on the scale, there is a pretty good chance that we will reach for whatever is closest and readily available, which is typically the packaged stuff. We can avoid doing this by *listening* to what our bodies are trying to tell us through our bodies' feedback loops.

Tune into your body's wisdom, and learn to pay attention to its signals.

Instead of taking it out on the kids when the hangry (combination of the word hungry and angry) side of you unleashes and you can't think clearly, it's important to listen to what the body is trying to convey through its signals.

It is essential to eat an actual meal instead of snacking constantly because the body will look for a meal until it receives it. But here's something else to consider: How will we know when we have had enough food? Most people eat until they feel so full they have to unbuckle their pants. If you are one of these people, what's another way you can tell the body has had enough food and you can prevent having to unbuckle? Chewing mindfully, eating slowly, and putting your fork down between bites will allow you to know when you are satisfied versus wolfing down the food in less than five minutes. It takes the body twenty minutes to know it is full, so stopping when you feel satisfied is the way to go.

When you are halfway through the meal, ask yourself how satisfied you are on a scale of 1 to 10. If you are at a 5, then keep this in mind so you do not get to a 10 and feel the need to unbuckle your pants. If you are not sure when you will feel satisfied, perhaps using the half-plate rule can help until you get the hang of things.

Half-Plate Rule

Half of your plate should consist of vegetables and one serving of a healthy fat (*not* saturated fat from meat). The other side of the plate is up to you. (Contrary to popular belief, you do not need to eat protein at every meal.) Superfoods like kale, hemp seeds, and almonds are a great way to get fiber, protein, and fat into a meal.

Once you are done, making a physical gesture such as pushing the plate away or crossing your silverware can signal the end of the meal.

Recommended Meal Times

According to the book *The Ayurveda Way* by Ananta Ripa Ajmera, Ayurveda recommends eating your largest meal around noon when the sun is the strongest and eating a small meal at dinner. All of

Ayurveda's daily practices are synced with the sun's cycle, and that's why Ayurveda recommends eating breakfast between seven and nine o'clock in the morning, lunch between noon and one-thirty in the afternoon, and dinner between five and seven o'clock in the evening. Keep at least three hours between meals in order for the previous meal to fully be digested to prevent digestive problems. Ajmera also recommends taking deep breaths before eating to calm the mind and body. Emotions are like food; if they aren't properly digested, they can harm your mind and body.

Self-Preservation

Self-preservation mode is a state in which the brain feels it needs to be in order to make sure that we live another day. This usually shows up in our thinking patterns, mental habits, and physical habits. For example, if I am the first car in line to go at a traffic light, counting two seconds before pressing the gas pedal after the traffic light turns green is a habit I have formed as a form of self-preservation to prevent hitting a driver who runs a red light.

The thing to question is whether the mental and physical habits are truly serving us or hurting us. When it comes to food, the brain knows it is essential for survival. But what the brain doesn't fully understand is which foods truly ensure our survival and which ones will end up hurting us or even killing us in the long run. Bringing awareness to how food impacts the body can help the brain link pain to certain foods and pleasure with others. We have all been programmed to think that sugar and sweets bring pleasure, and they do for a minute, but what about after that minute?

My Miserable Habit Loop

Every Monday, I would make a mental commitment to avoid eating anything with sugar for the rest of the week. But I would always take the easy way out and give in, eat the sugary thing I saw, feel good for a minute, feel guilty about not sticking to my commitment, and then feel miserable physically and mentally. But then I would tell myself to step up and make next Monday the true start date. Then I decided to stick in a cheat day, but that made things even worse. My brain believed that I could not break this cycle because this is how I would stay alive, and my *belief* was that I wasn't strong enough to break free from it, so I kept doing this for years. But not anymore. My Tony Robbins results coach Traci Butz helped me break free from this habit loop and see myself in a new way—a more powerful way. The new version of me is committed to making health a priority. If you are willing to make health a priority in your life, anything is possible.

During my journey, I learned that there's a difference between guilt and shame. Shame is when you feel bad, broken, or unworthy. It happens when you tell yourself lies and believe them. Guilt, on the other hand, is remorse for something you have done. It can actually be a constructive emotion, empowering you to make important behavioral shifts. Just as a plant needs water, sunshine, and care to grow, our minds need similar nurturing. Based on this new perspective from Ajmera's book *The Ayurveda Way*, I have been able to bring a greater sense of awareness to different aspects of my life and build upon that awareness constructively.

Sugar Habit Tracker

The first step in breaking free from the sugar habit is to *become aware* of when you reach for sugar because habits are usually actions done without much thought. Building awareness will build self-knowledge and improve self-regulation.

Over the course of three to six days (six days is recommended), track when you reach for something with sugar *and* artificial sweeteners from the time you wake up to the time you go to sleep on the Sugar Habit Tracker.

Please write down the time of day and food or beverage you consume. Once this is done, check to see if you have a sugar habit by circling any patterns you notice. That's it for now.

As you progress through this book, the upcoming BAM moments will explain what to do using the information gathered on the chart. But just as a heads-up, the next step will be to focus your attention on *one* habit you would like to shift. You must then *find a replacement* for the habit.

If you don't want to carry around a piece of paper and a pen to note your sugar habits, you could put notes in your phone or take photos of the foods and drinks or be creative and find a way that works for you. I would not recommend relying on your memory because you may not remember everything or may purposely block things out of your memory. We've all been there. Then find a little bit of time to write things down so you can see it in front of you as a chart and look for patterns and note the habits. It may surprise you how many times you reach for sugar.

A blank tracker is available in Appendix A, or it can be downloaded from my website. If printing the sheets are not possible, simply draw three columns on two separate sheets of paper.

So your morning coffee with sugar or tea with honey would be on this list.

Sugar Habit Tracker

The first step in breaking free from the sugar habit is to **become aware** of when you consume sugar.

Write down the time of day and food or drink that has sugar or artificial sweeteners over the course of 3 to 6 days. Once this is done, circle any patterns you notice.

Note: If printing this sheet from my website is not possible, simply draw 3 columns on a sheet of paper.

Day 1	Day 2	Day 3

<u>Sugar Habit Tracker</u>

Please continue to write down the time of day and food or drink that has sugar or artificial sweeteners. Once this is done, check to see if you have a sugar habit by circling any repetitive patterns you notice.

Day 4	Day 5	Day 6

Things that you didn't think have sugar actually do, such as the sauce and cheese on a pizza and the salad dressing (that's why people feel hungry even after eating a gigantic salad with the works). So the big question is: What am I supposed to eat? Everything has sugar! We'll tackle that later. For now, just focus on jotting down things that you eat that have sugar. If you are out and can't look at the ingredient list, jot it down if you think it might have sugar or artificial sweeteners.

Do you start the day with a muffin and tea with honey? (Sugar is just about always one of the first three ingredients in muffins.) Is that something you would like to change?

The key to habit change will be to make small almost unnoticeable *shifts.*

Habit change could start with a change as small as putting in one less spoon of sugar into your coffee just like my husband. He is no longer Mr. Grouchy, which is a great thing for everyone in the family.

In the book *Making Habits, Breaking Habits*, Jeremy Dean states that habit change is not a sprint. It's a marathon. You must get into this mindset. Make one small change that you can replicate every day until you don't know that you are not doing it anymore. And then move onto to the next habit. Trying to change more than one thing at a time will work for a little while, but just like diet fads, it will stop working. So if you are truly committed to lifting yourself up, commit to a small act and believe that you can do it. Take on the mindset of an explorer and enjoy the journey!

Dean also states that habits are automatically activated by our environments, and most people eat at the same place every day and stick to the same foods. This type of habit has led to staggering statistics. Since 1980, the number of overweight people has doubled, and the number of obese people has quadrupled.

= Brain Activation Mode = BAM

Pinpoint *one* habit you would like to shift. It's really important to only focus on *one* habit. Trying to change too many things at once will lead to frustration.

After you have chosen your habit, pinpoint exactly when it happens. Is it every weekday morning? At night on weekends?

So now that you have decided, ask yourself these questions: *Do I want to keep doing this?* and *How does this help or hurt me?*

If your answer to the first question, "Do I want to keep doing this?" was an emphatic no, then that's a favorable habit to target right now. If it was a yes or a maybe, then please choose a different one; otherwise, you won't put enough effort into it. It must feel like it's important for you to shift the habit.

If your answer to the second question, "How does this help me or hurt me?" was, "This isn't helping me at all because I feel like a train hit me by the end of the day," or, "My head feels like it's going to explode," then that might be the habit to target.

Think possibilities.

Find an Empowering Alternative

Because old habits must be replaced with new habits, make sure that the new habit is an empowering one. By that I mean that replacing eating with smoking is not going to empower you. But replacing eating with looking outside and taking deep breaths while looking at the clouds passing by will empower you by making you live more in the present. This may seem like a small act, but it is actually huge on the psyche. If this isn't your cup of tea, at least clouds are free versus cigarettes, which will take a toll on your wallet. Instead of spending money on carcinogens, every time you are tempted to buy something sugary, add that amount to an excel sheet on your phone. Once it adds up to quite a bit, buy something you have always wanted like a Fitbit or take a trip and let that be your escape. Even though external rewards are not the best approach, perhaps this will get things started, and you will amass the energy needed for your trip.

Things to Do in the Moment

My habit substitution list included:

- Take deep breaths and say a power statement. (Mine is, "My quality of life depends on eating quality foods.")
- Eat a handful of nuts.
- Smell or drink tea. (Sometimes just smelling it is enough for me. Tazo and Rishi make some divine-smelling teas. Gymnema sylvestre is a natural herb that can be found in tea, and it is designed to stave off food cravings. It really works!)
- Sip or gulp down a cup of water.

= Brain Activation Mode = BAM

What might your habit substitution list consist of? What can you do instead that would help make you feel better?"

Which one of the choices will help you take care of your body?

Pinpoint *one* alternative that will make you feel equally fulfilled or more fulfilled than the previous habit.

Once you have decided on the habit, you must make a commitment to stick with it and do it *consistently* in place of the previous habit.

Think possibilities.

Breaking Free from Mental Habits

If you'd like to change a mental habit rather than a physical habit such as feeling sorry for yourself before eating, constantly criticizing yourself, resisting cravings and then giving in, or feeling shame and guilt after eating something, you just need to take the same steps as a physical habit.

You need to pinpoint *one* habit and substitute it with an empowering alternative. The alternative must be done consistently to build in automaticity.

For instance, let's say you eat a piece of sugary food when you come home in the evening, and then you tell yourself that you are weak and that you will never be strong enough to do anything good in life. Replacing the habit of putting yourself down with brushing your teeth will take away the time and space for your brain to go into negative self-talk mode and make you get out of your head and take action. Afterward, you could go read or listen to a book like *The Universe Has Your Back* by Gabrielle Bernstein to make you feel empowered.

The key to habit change is changing your emotional state and your physiology, according to Tony Robbins. So going from criticizing yourself to brushing your teeth or something energizing like a push-up against the wall will change your mental and physical state. Replacing the negative self-talk with positive self-talk will, of course, be very helpful.

Curiosity, Consistency, and Compassion

In order to be able to create a new habit, there are 3 C's to keep in mind:

- Curiosity
- Consistency
- Compassion

Curiosity

Studies show that being mean to ourselves doesn't help; it actually hurts us. However, being curious can help, and this can be interpreted in different ways. It can mean asking questions about what's happening in the moment and being mindful of life here and now. Using the senses to be mindful and curious activates the pleasure parts of the brain and allows the body to be in a state of rest rather than stress. Curiosity invites us to stop focusing on the end result. It makes us meet things as they are and appreciate progress. Focusing on something in the moment allows us to let go of the reactive mind and the need to control everything and moves us to the responsive mind that knows how to make kind and skillful choices, according to the book *The Gift of our Compulsions* by Mary O'Malley.

Consistency

Consistency is the key to breaking free from an old habit. You must be consistent with the new habit in order to build in the automaticity.

Compassion

Being nice to yourself and being compassionate through positive self-talk can increase confidence and self-regulation. An increase in self-control can lead to less impulsive actions and the ability to make better choices. According to O'Malley, the opposite of control is not being out of control. Rather, it is about bringing curiosity, clarity, and compassion to whatever you are experiencing. As kids, we were taught how to ride a bike and read but not how to be okay with ourselves. Eventually, the judging and comparing of ourselves to others causes pain, and the brain tries to find a way to deal with the pain in disempowering ways. But we can turn that around and accept ourselves for who we are and where we are.

Breaking free from a habit can be hard, especially if it's something you have done for years. But habits are not impossible to outgrow. However, if you do think it's impossible, you've got to revisit and revise your belief; otherwise, the brain will not rewire itself.

If you do end up giving in, be gentle with yourself and acknowledge that it will take time. At this point in the book, the habit-changing process is happening at the surface level, kind of like building something with Legos. I invite you to continue reading the book and learning ways to make the new habit stick by going below the surface and building your ride with the toughest stuff out there so it becomes tough enough to withstand anything.

For instance, let's say that you have a habit of always saying yes to people. If someone offers you a sugary thing, you always say yes even though you don't want it. If we invite curiosity to shed some light on this habit, digging deeper would entail wondering where the need to please everyone comes from.

At the surface level, if saying the word *no* is hard to muster up, instead of always saying yes, you could say, "I'm good for now," or, "Maybe later." When it comes to habits, how you do one thing is how you do everything. If saying no to food is hard, then chances are saying no to other things in your life is hard too. So you pack your schedule with a million things because you keep saying yes to everyone, get overwhelmed, and wonder why everyone keeps depending on you for so many things.

Establishing boundaries and acknowledging that you can't be everything for everyone all the time begins with scheduling time for self-care. This, in turn, will help you and others in the long run.

Self-Care Can Lead to Feelings of Empowerment

I would recommend creating a list of nourishing activities that allows you to do some ultimate self-care, like getting a foot massage (reflexology can really do wonders), taking a stroll, going to a comedy club and laughing your head off (laughter really is the best medicine), or meditating. Make it a time to rejuvenate the soul, so you can become stronger. Self-care or self-kindness is a form of empowerment. It is not a form of selfishness.

Self-care could also mean taking a minute to be grateful for the things in your life like the sun, the moon, or a warm bed. People who are grateful for things in their lives, their families, or their jobs do not want to hurt themselves. A grateful heart truly is a happy heart.

Taking the time to take care of ourselves allows us to recognize and honor our feelings. By being more aware and present, we're in a better position to be a more compassionate spouse, parent, coworker, friend, and human being.

I once had the privilege of hearing Dr. Sean Stephenson, otherwise known as the three-foot giant, speak at a conference. He said that if you focus on what you don't have, you are going to be miserable. What do you want out of life? He said asking this will give you the energy and power to shift the focus from fear to excitement.

He went on to say that he chose to be in the body he is in, even though he has had to endure a lot of hardship given that sneezing could break his ribs due to his rare bone disease. But he said something really profound that resonated with a lot of us in the audience. He quoted someone who once said, "Pain is inevitable. Suffering is optional."

Giving up a habit will feel painful, especially if you feel that it is part of your identity. So if it is not a habit you want to change quite yet, you might want to consider a different one.

But if you are ready to cut down or abstain from drinking wine, at first you might miss it because you have always thought of yourself as a wine sommelier and you can no longer be one. Or perhaps drinking wine is special because it's one of the few things you do with your spouse and you will miss the special time together. So what could you do?

In some ways, it can be hard to overlook the things you are losing, especially if it's part of your identity. Saying goodbye to old habits and ways of being and your old self can be a lot to bear, but it means you can be stronger and give more than before. Here is an opportunity to step up and show up for yourself.

Perhaps pouring in less wine will help with the transition. If you drink two glasses, cut down to one and a half and then to one and so on. Essentially, you would reduce the amount gradually or go from daily to fewer days a week. Perhaps the wine could eventually be substituted with a cup of an aromatic herbal tea or a really great book.

Focus on What Your Body Will Be Able to *Do*

Another way to decide which habit to hone in on is to choose one that will allow your body to do something it couldn't do before. Rather than focusing on how your body will *look* different, focus on what your body will be able to *do* and *accomplish* with the habit change. So if you don't seem to have the energy to go outside and walk around the block, decrease the amount of sugar you eat at night, especially before bed, so you can wake up with more energy. Before you go to work or drop the kids off at school, walk to the end of your driveway, take a deep breath, tell yourself you did it, and then walk back toward your house. Small steps literally and figuratively are the key to permanent habit change.

Focusing on one habit and being consistent with it will help you gain the resiliency you need to keep on going. There is no such thing as failure. If you try something and it doesn't work, try something else. Send those positive vibes to the universe that you can do this, and you will be surprised on how a positive mindset can change your outlook on things. Removing the word *fail* from your vocabulary might help do the trick as well.

Text message to the universe: What is something you would like to *do* that you can't do now?

CHAPTER 5

How Do I Spot Triggers and Set Anchors?

CLEAR your mind of the word can't and replace it with I CAN.

So what is a trigger or a cue exactly? How does it set us off and possibly sabotage us? It could be something we see, hear, smell, taste, or touch that causes some sort of reaction. It somehow triggers a *need* to do something even if we don't understand why, and we feel compelled to follow through with whatever it may be. When I worked in the Office of Teacher Education at Teachers College, I used to be in the habit of turning my neck to the left when I entered the reception area to see if there was any free food sitting on the kitchen counter. There would usually be all sorts of sugary stuff that people either brought in or was left over from an event. Then I realized that seeing the food there was a trigger for me, so I stopped turning my neck to the left and just kept my eyes straight toward my office. Believe it not, this helped a lot. The first few times were not so hard because there was nothing there anyway, but then hearing people talk about how delicious something was in the kitchen made me wonder if I should go take a peek. But then I got into the habit of drinking water and telling myself not to confuse thirst with hunger and that it was not mealtime, so I shouldn't eat anything. This took several weeks to achieve because I went from eating every one to two hours to eating every three to four hours. It may not seem like that big of a difference, but if you try doing this, you'll see that the confusing thirst with hunger thing can easily go out the door. I would allow myself food if I was physically feeling dizzy or feeling hunger pains. But if it was purely mental, I just tried to focus on my work, or I would go find someone to talk to distract me.

There will be triggers everywhere. How do they show up in our lives? When do they show up? Some triggers can't be removed easily, so what options do we have to work around them?

When you see something that triggers you, acknowledge that it's there. Acknowledgment is the first step to building awareness.

A fellow health coach by the name of Heidi Hochstetler, founder of HZH Coaching, told me an interesting story about going to the mall with her sisters when she was younger. Since shopping together didn't happen frequently, it was a special experience, and the day would always end with a huge sunda__ at Friendly's. They never left the mall without going there. To her, this was an endearing experience: a time to be together.

As an adult, Heidi took her own daughters on a shopping trip and spotted a Friendly's restaurant. She bought them the same sunda__ she had as a kid. Seeing the Friendly's triggered her to do something special with her daughters even though she didn't want them to eat it because of the high sugar content. But her brain must have associated the sunda__ with feelings of love, safety, and belonging. In an attempt to *re-create* those feelings, Heidi felt compelled to buy the sunda_ even though she didn't want to get it. They couldn't finish it, and they didn't really enjoy it. Heidi now recognizes that seeing a Friendly's was a trigger and that there are other ways to spend quality time with family.

One of the few childhood memories I have around food involves going to the supermarket with my parents and filling up the cart with every type of junk food imaginable. When we got to the register, we would play a game to see who could match the total cost of everything in the cart to the receipt. I realize now that I used to do the same thing when my kids were younger. I would encourage them to use their sense of exploration to seek out and put colorful boxes and treats in the cart, so they could be happy. But I seriously regret that now because instead of making them happy, I was making them sick. But I have learned from my past mistakes, and now a trip to the supermarket with the kids includes one item of choice if it doesn't have sugar listed as one of the first three ingredients in addition to one fruit of choice and one new vegetable to try.

When we come home, I try to get them to help make the meal that includes the vegetable they chose. This provides them with a sense of ownership over the dish they created, and they are much more likely to enjoy the meal.

Invisible Triggers

Stress and emotions are the invisible triggers that play a big part in the reward- and comfort-seeking mission by the brain. Instead of seeking that instant relief, empower yourself by bringing awareness to the thoughts and feelings you are experiencing. According to McGonigal, knowing *what they are* can be empowering.

I spent years trying to distract myself in every way possible and seek out something other than food to fulfill that mission, but I learned that distractions can only go so far. Once I became aware of these triggers, acknowledged them, accepted them, felt them, and let go of them, I finally started to make progress.

American society looks down on people who are emotional or can't cope with stress well, and it tells people that eating food for comfort is the way to go. But it's time to change the messaging. Emotions are what makes us human. We should be allowed to feel emotions and show them instead of hiding them and eating food to cover them up.

Instead of allowing triggers to rule us and have power over us, converting the trigger into an anchor means we have mastered habit change.

Anticipation can give you a huge advantage in life, in sports, at work, and just about anywhere. *Anticipating* triggers is the *key*. Wayne Gretzky is known for being one of greatest ice hockey players of all time because he went to where the puck was going. If you don't anticipate, you could end up facing frustration and pain. If you can eventually turn triggers that made you weak into something that makes you strong, you can reach a level of personal mastery like no other.

= Brain Activation Mode = BAM

Please take a moment to think about triggers in your environment or invisible triggers that cause you to reach for sugar or cause you to do something you don't want to do.

What sets you off? What is it that you have a hard time saying no to?

What are some action steps that you can take to work around them? Doing some "If … then …" planning has shown to boost success rates up to three times, according to Mel Robbins in her book *The 5 Second Rule*.

Think of a trigger—what could be an "if … then …" plan for that trigger?

For example: *If* I see a can of soda, *then* I will walk away and congratulate myself for not drinking it.

Think possibilities.

= Beyond BAM =

If you try to get into a mindful mindset, asking yourself, "Where is my need coming from?" might lead to some surprising answers.

What am I attaching it to?

Is it supposed to solve a problem?

What emotions am I attaching to this food?

Why do I eat it even though I don't really want it or need it?

Becoming aware of triggers is crucial to rewiring a habit because it expands our awareness of why we do what we do.

Anchors and Accountability

Symbolically, anchors represent stability and strength, so we want to set some down to ground us and keep us steady. Anchors can take on many shapes and forms. The more creative they are, the better!

Below of some examples of anchors I have used:

- Visual: Signs that say, "Find your light," and, "My quality of life depends on eating quality food," on a bathroom mirror or screensaver
- Audio: Songs such as "Have It All" by Jason Mraz and "Fight Song" by Rachel Platten
- Taste: Peppermint tea and chamomile tea
- Smell: Eucalyptus oil and stress-relief blends
- Touch: Lavender oil

I would recommend instituting an anchor using at least three of the five senses around your home, office, car, or anywhere that you go daily.

> **Anchors can also hold us accountable for our actions and act as friendly reminders to keep going in the face of big, sugary monsters in our faces.**

Text message to the universe: What anchors can you put down to keep you grounded?

CHAPTER 6

How Do I Break Free from My Patterns?

Stop looking around for permission from other people to be amazing.
—Sean Stephenson

Our subconscious minds have a way to control our patterns in ways that we are not aware of, but making ourselves conscious of these patterns by bringing awareness to them can change our entire landscape and start the breakthrough process. Once we become aware of the pieces of the pattern, we can become aware of how our *emotions* can either lift our view of life or disassemble our lives. So you might say, "I have a tendency to overeat." Your behavior will lead to your result, which will be to become overweight. But what's behind all of this? According to Tony Robbins, it's an *emotional pattern or state of mind* that makes you behave this way. So changing the behavior is not going to change the emotion because you will still feel the same way and look for an outlet.

So what should we do? If you catch yourself feeling sad at the end of the day, acknowledge this emotion. Then use either your body, voice, or focus to interrupt it and do something different than what you always do. Do something totally off the grid if you can. If you always go to the pantry and take out the sugary stuff as soon as you get home because this is what you are programmed to do, interrupt the pattern by blasting music and singing. Allow for a different type of release to settle in. Interrupting old, limiting patterns and creating new, more empowering alternatives and conditioning these is the secret to lasting change, according to Tony Robbins.

Pinpointing Emotional Patterns

If you would like to find the emotional pattern, I would recommend using the Sugar Habit Tracker again, but this time *note the emotion you feel before* eating the *food you are craving* for six days.

After the six days, circle patterns and try to pinpoint the trigger that causes you to feel this way, consider how to work around the trigger, and look for ways to change the behavior and work through the emotion.

Scramble the Pattern

Pretend you are coloring in a picture of a Ferris wheel and staying inside the lines. Now go crazy with the crayon until you can't see the image anymore. That's how much scrambling needs to take place. Going out of the lines a couple of times is not going to make the picture look all scrambled. You've got to put in some effort and commit to scratching out what was underneath. This is essentially what you are doing when you turn on the music instead of eating the sugary food.

We create our own miseries. Because we create them, we have the power to dispel them. It's our choice. We can sit there and stew over the fact that someone hurt our feelings, *or* we can learn from it and tell ourselves that next time we hear negative words, we will tell ourselves that everyone is entitled to their own opinion and say a mantra such as, "Life will get better."

Let's look at the previous example from a different angle. You have come home and feel sad and ashamed because of the way your home looks. We become habituated to what we have, so we must be careful to compare and contrast things in an empowering way. If your house lacks furniture or is small or is dark and rundown and you dread going to it, comparing it to the houses of coworkers or friends is not going to help in any way. So what can help?

Ask yourself this question: What can help make me feel better about coming home?

Perhaps it could be something as simple as adding a splash of color by finding or writing some inspirational sayings such as, "Positive thoughts bring positive things," or "Nothing can stop the miracles heading my way."

I have many pictures of lotus flowers all over my office because it amazes me how something so beautiful can come from a dark and muddy place. Looking at the lotus inspires me, and it brings such a beautiful touch of color to the room.

Many people underestimate the importance of their environments. The environmental factors around us can either act as triggers or anchors for our moods and feelings. Opening the shade and curtains in the morning and looking at the sky can lift up our mood instantly.

The Imperfect Mindset

The book *How to Be an Imperfectionist* by Stephen Guise discusses perfectionism as an invisible habit. It's a systematic way of thinking that holds us back in a lot of negative ways. Perfectionism frequently leads to people being depressed because reality is a disaster in comparison to their perfect expectations. Guise sheds light on how being a perfectionist is not really a strength when it comes to our perception of the world, but it is rather an illusion of greatness. We do this by living passively and watching television for hours on end or doing some other type of numbing activity because it is automatic, rewarding, and mistake-free. Guise also points out that what he describes as "self-handicapping" holds us back by making up a million excuses for not achieving something, such as a knee that hurts or tiredness, so if we don't give it our all, there's an excuse why it wasn't the best it could have been. So how can we take bold strides instead of tiptoeing?

For lasting change to occur, the brain must create new neural pathways through the three Cs: *curiosity, consistency,* and *compassion.* If this doesn't happen, the old patterns and ways will resurface.

Mixed Neuro-Associations

Mixed neuro-associations occur when the brain associates pain and pleasure to something at the same time, according to a blog post by Team Tony. This makes the brain go into overload, and it gets really confused, which can lead to poor decision-making. When I realized that this is what was happening to my brain and I could finally put a name to it, I was thrilled beyond belief.

When this happens, Tony Robbins recommends writing down the pros and cons of your potential decision and weighing them out to help search for a solution. Decide which ones are valid and which ones are misperceptions. Then decide which ones really matter to you. Doing this should help move forward with the better choice.

If you find that you continuously make poor choices, it might be because you don't have a big enough why or reason attached for doing what you are doing. This was a huge aha moment for me in my conversation with my results coach. I had a ton of reasons why I should stop eating sugar, but I didn't have a *big* enough reason *why* because even though I didn't feel well after I ate it, the truth is I still found pleasure in eating it.

Abstainers and Moderators

I tried really, really hard to completely eliminate sugar for more than a few weeks at a time, but my attempt to be perfect was causing me a lot of stress and frustration. Then I came upon Gretchen Rubin's book *Better Than Before*, where she talks about abstainers and moderators. Abstainers are people who have to keep their distance from sugar and keep it out of their system completely. On the other hand, moderators can eat sugary stuff in moderation, and it won't escalate unlike abstainers where one cook__ becomes two, which then becomes three, four, and so on. For abstainers, having something makes them want it more; for moderators, having something makes them want it less.

Cravings are provoked by possibility rather than by denial.

A general rule of thumb is if you eat fewer sweets, you will crave fewer sweets.

If you can't decide whether you would be better off as an abstainer or moderator, Rubin suggests asking yourself this question: If you eat one square of choc__ on a choc___ bar, are you fine, or do you end up wanting more? If you are fine, you are a moderator. If not, you are better off abstaining and saving your willpower for other, more important decisions. Eventually, deprivation no longer becomes an issue because you don't feel like you are missing out on anything. Abstainers do better when they follow all-or-nothing habits, according to Rubin.

Another way to think of it is through a paradigm shift by moving from:

I want that, but I can't have it.

to

I *can* have it, but I don't want it.

Reframing Sugar Intake

My rules around sugar changed with every passing week, month, and season. I was always looking for exceptions and loopholes so I could eat sugar. I decided that I was going to stick to one simple rule: Don't eat anything with sugar. Who was I kidding?! Then after eating a little bit of this and that to see if it escalated and I wanted more, I decided to allow myself sugar under these circumstances: 1) The ingredient list has vegetables, and sugar is at the bottom of the list (like the veggie cakes sold at Costco), and 2) When I am on vacation or traveling. If I only have one chance to try a particular food, I will take that opportunity because access to it is not easy. I am more at peace with food now that I allow myself sugar under these situations. I no longer fight cravings, and this has led to much more peaceful outcomes.

After trying to eat in moderation many times, I have found that the only way to deal with the cravings is to do the inner work and have my heart and mind tell me that I am better off without it. Studies show that people who show more compassion toward themselves are better able to cope and be more resilient, while people who are full of self-blame struggle more.

Text message to the universe: Do you see yourself as a moderator or an abstainer or neither?

2
PART

HOW TO USE AWARENESS TO IMPROVE YOUR QUALITY OF LIFE

CHAPTER 7

How Can I Tell How Food Impacts My Body?

Start where you are. Use what you have. Do what you can.
—Arthur Ashe

If you have ever been on a real roller coaster and did not enjoy it, you probably felt nauseous or achy afterward. The impact on your body was very obvious, very fast.

On the symbolic roller coaster, the impact could occur within minutes, within one to two hours, be delayed by seventy-two hours, or stay hidden for several years or decades.

My father used to drink a powdered blend of mixed grains and nuts with hot water every morning. He would feel blood rushing to his head within minutes, and it made him feel very dizzy. He never thought to consider that what he thought was a healthy blend was affecting his body in a negative way. But once he became aware of this, he reduced the amount of the mixture in each serving and eventually stopped drinking it.

Small changes begin with awareness.

How the Body Communicates with Us

The collection of visceral fat, especially along the midline and face, are common when it comes to the overconsumption of sugar. Visceral fat builds up around the organs, so it becomes harder for organs such as the liver and pancreas to work properly, which leads to health problems like type 2 diabetes.

To all the men out there: beer bellies are a big sign of an imbalance in the body. All of the stored fat sitting in the midline is a huge red flag and a possible sign of a pending heart attack or stroke. Red flags require attention.

Another obvious way to tell if sugar is hurting you is through the mouth. Tooth decay and cavities are soaring through the roof. It was heartbreaking to watch a documentary called *Is Sugar the New Fat?* and seeing a two-year-old getting six of her rotten teeth pulled out. She will not only have problems eating at that age, but her orthodontic problems will be something she will have to deal with in adulthood as well. Sugary drinks like juice and soda are the biggest culprits of tooth decay.

There are many other ways to notice the impact of refined foods. Do you sometimes feel forgetful and wonder why you can't remember something? It could be the impact of a meal that you ate that was high in refined carbohydrates or wheat flour. Believe it or not, things like forgetfulness can impact your brain as quickly as you ate the sandwich.

My husband would sometimes give my son a hard time about not remembering to do something right after he was told to do so like picking up things that were on the floor. But after reading an article about the effects of fast food on the body, I realized that it wasn't totally my son's disregard for cleaning up after himself. It was his brain and the food he'd just eaten. Ever since he'd started at his new school, he had been eating a slice of pizza or chicken nuggets for lunch every day. Those are some of the worst foods to eat—pizza has sugar, and who knows what's in the nuggets. I have asked him to buy some vegetables to accompany the meal, but apparently the lettuce is wilted and the fruit is not appealing or sitting in syrup. It's no wonder kids are not able to focus in school and behavioral problems are an issue.

Breakfast has been said to be one of the most important meals of the day, but it is actually one of the worst in terms of food because sugary cereals, sweet pastries, or processed meats like bacon usually make up the standard American breakfast. All of which are what the body does *not* need, especially first thing in the morning. So what should people eat? It's time to go to the supermarket and start looking for almonds or different varieties of hummus, like everything bagel hummus. I like to soak almonds in water for at least an hour before eating them in order to soften them. Or just skip breakfast. People can live on two meals a day. Eat an early lunch if possible, as well as an early dinner so that no more than four to six hours pass between meals. My husband went from eating a bagel every morning to eating nothing in the morning, and he feels much better. Find what works for you and your body.

Intermittent Fasting

Intermittent fasting can be a healthy lifestyle with many benefits, according to Dr. Jason Fung. He has helped cure thousands of people who had type 2 diabetes and cancer through fasting regimens. If cancer cells don't have anything toxic to feed off of in the body, they can't live. Thus, removing toxic foods for long periods of time can cure many illnesses and is a great preventative measure as well.

Effects of Sugar

Many people in the United States are overfed yet starving of nutrients at the cellular level because of food choices. In order to study the impact of food on our bodies, we need a method of measurement. We can do this by measuring our energy level, gassiness, headaches, or something else that causes us discomfort or pain.

Below is a list of ways sugar could impact the body. Choose at least one or two things from the list that you have had to deal with currently or in the recent past to gauge how your body is being impacted by food choices:

Physical Effects

- Blurred vision/loss of vision
- Headaches
- Tooth decay
- Bad breath
- Body odor
- Skin issues—acne or eczema
- Premature aging—wrinkles or saggy skin
- Unstable energy levels
- Gassiness—belching or flatulence
- Digestive distress—indigestion
- Bloating
- Fatigue
- Increased thirst
- Gout/joint pain
- Asthma-type symptoms
- Constipation
- Impotency in men

- Painful and heavy menstrual cycles in women
- Frequent urination—overactive bladder
- Weak immune system—frequent colds
- Worsening of allergies
- Weight gain

Mental Effects

- Depression
- Mood swings
- Hyperactivity
- Sleepiness
- Intense cravings
- Difficulty concentrating—brain fog
- Memory impairment—forgetfulness or dementia
- Aggressiveness (more likely in males)
- Anxiety—panic attacks, nervousness, constant worrying, restlessness, tension (more likely in females)

Hidden Effects

Then there are the less obvious but profound effects that build over time, such as heart disease, diabetes, fatty liver, kidney disease, rheumatoid arthritis, osteoporosis, cancer, and other autoimmune diseases.

= Brain Activation Mode = BAM

What will be your methods of measurement?

How and how often will you assess how your body is doing?

For example, if you chose gassiness and bloating as your methods of measurement because you have been experiencing those things recently, make a note or send a text message to yourself that you kept burping after eating your ham sandwich and that you felt really bloated after eating a big bowl of pineapples. Please keep some sort of record of your reactions to food over the next two weeks or more.

After each week, take a look at how often you didn't feel well and what foods caused those reactions. Try to be more mindful if you eat them again and make attempts to choose a better alternative.

Think possibilities.

So you've read about how food impacts the body immediately. Now I want to share another way: the next morning.

Body Scan Log

When you wake up and open your eyes, before you even get out of bed, take a minute to do a body scan. Start at the top of the head and check in to see how you feel. Does your head feel achy, heavy, or lightheaded? Then go to the eyes. Do you feel pressure behind the eyes? Does your nose feel stuffy? Does the inside of your mouth feel pasty or dry? Check in with the rest of your body and continue with your neck, shoulders, back, arms, belly, legs, and feet. Take one to two minutes to do this, and you might be surprised with what you notice.

Then see how much energy you have to get out of bed. If you feel lethargic, it's a sign that your body has come to a big crash. If you want to stop feeling this way, you've got to get off the sugar roller coaster and balance your glucose levels.

Make this part of your morning routine for at least two weeks.

Once you start to associate pain or discomfort with sugar or another food you are eating, your brain will want to stay away from it.

CHAPTER 8

How Will I Know If My Body Is Getting Better?

Your body hears everything your mind says. Stay positive.

Some benefits can be felt in two days, two weeks, four weeks, or more depending on how much sugar you used to consume. If you consumed small amounts, you probably won't go through too many withdrawal symptoms. But you might experience withdrawal symptoms for up to two weeks or possibly longer before you start to shine if you consumed a lot of sugar. Withdrawal symptoms could include headaches, dizziness, fatigue, and flu-like symptoms, but don't get discouraged. Just keep telling yourself that this too shall pass, and brighter skies will show up once the dark clouds part.

Assessing Progress

If you have found your groove and feel powerful that you can maintain your new habit, consider removing more of the sugars to see even more benefits.

If you have not been able to be consistent in replacing your previous habit with your new habit, ask yourself what is stopping you from doing so. What are you believing to be true about yourself?

I was believing that I was not capable of committing to giving up sweets. It is still something I am working on, and the mindfulness practices in chapter 18 have really helped me work through shifting my old beliefs.

Huge Accomplishments May Seem Minor

Next time you reach for the ice cr__m in the freezer, if you hesitate for even one second, it means you are shifting your mental habits, and it is something worth celebrating. If it is no longer something you do without a second thought, and now it has become something that does require a second thought. That is *huge*!

Think about what you will be gaining as a result of the habit change rather than what you will be losing.

Getting the serotonin going in your gut and brain for little and big gains is really important to make new habits stick.

= Brain Activation Mode = BAM

How can you make sure you celebrate the little and big gains?

Think possibilities.

Text message to the universe: How will you know your body is getting better?

CHAPTER 9

Is Eating Sugar Just a Habit, or Could It Be an Addiction?

If you are depressed you are living in the past.
If you are anxious you are living in the future.
If you are at peace you are living in the present.
—Lao Tzu

The idea of having a sugar addiction can be kind of out there. The idea of being addicted to anything is not something people really want to boast about, but bringing awareness that this condition exists is the first step. Addictions are usually a *symptom* of something, according to a speech by Tony Robbins. It's not about finding the root or cause of the symptom, which can take years of therapy. Looking for patterns and breaking them is what makes the difference because it sets off a chain of events. According to Robbins, it's more about finding the *source*. Which of the six needs are not being met that makes people seek out something destructive?

The *craving* for a little something is your body's way of communicating to you that it needs energy, whether it is emotional energy or another type of energy. According to Ayurveda, cravings for sweets are usually cravings for love, connection, and belonging.

If you believe that you are not capable of turning things around and think of yourself as weak and powerless, then that's where you'll likely stay, unfortunately. Trying to find the motivation to change can be tricky because it can be hard to generate even with the best of intentions. Even if we have it, it usually doesn't last beyond six weeks before it starts to dissipate, and we go back to the old ways.

So why should we remove something that brings us comfort when we don't seem to get very much of it already? I invite you to focus on a new type of feeling, such as empowerment. Replacing feelings of guilt and shame with power and resilience could lead to accomplishing something you didn't even know you could do.

In some cases, a severe trauma or abuse might be the underlying reason for self-medicating through food. There are many reasons why people may seek solace through food, but if you are ready to make positive changes in your life, there is a quote in the Louise Hay "How to Love Yourself Cards" box that says, "When I am ready to make positive changes in my life, I attract whatever I need to help me."

Louise Hay, a famous motivational author, was abused at a young age and endured many different types of abuse for many years. She believed that the guilt and shame from all of those traumatic events manifested themselves physically through cancer in her body. Rather than seeking Western treatment through chemotherapy, she opted to do a mental and physical cleansing through the removal of factory-made foods, reflexology, and other holistic approaches. Within six months, she was cured of her cancer. It is hard to believe that this could happen, but our beliefs are the key to making progress. What we believe about ourselves is what drives us. Louise Hay believed that she could conquer her illness her own way, and her belief led to her decisions, which led to her ultimate outcome: a mind free of shame and guilt, and one that was filled with forgiveness and compassion, as well as a body free of disease, and one that was healed and clean.

There is no age limit for transformations to occur. Louise Hay was fifty years old when she published her first book *Heal Your Body*, and she went on to write a second book titled *You Can Heal Your Life*, which has changed the lives of millions of people around the world. I became a believer that the mind can heal the body after reading her story and her book.

Conquering Sugar Addiction with the Help of a Coach

A dysfunctional reward system fueled by wanting to feel better can lead to addictions. An addiction is anything that interferes with everyday life, stops people from being productive, and prevents people from being in the right headspace. This is what my results coach Traci Butz from the Tony Robbins Results Coaching Program pointed out to me in my first session. The need to feel good by eating sugary things is one thing. Obsessing over it and not giving up on getting it is another. I would obsess over getting that sweet something for days until I finally got my hands on it. I knew this was an issue, but I never thought of myself as an addict. Identifying myself as an addict was difficult to swallow. But once I realized and accepted this about myself, I knew what I had to do to conquer it. I felt committed to getting rid of those old ways because I kept telling myself that health is my priority, not putting food in my mouth. The need for sweet treats was wrecking my life, but I couldn't stop.

My coach pointed out that there are two sides of me: there is the Julia who wants to be productive and control the urges, and there is the sugar-addicted side that wants instant relief from what I am feeling in the moment.

I had been underplaying what was happening to me and thought it was just an issue of delayed gratification versus instant gratification until delaying it made me so miserable that my quality of life started to go downhill. I stopped seeing life in a positive way full of gratitude and started seeing things as awful and full of loneliness. I had trained my brain to crave this drug, so to speak, and in order to break free from the misery, I had to convince my brain that I was better off without it.

I had to find a replacement for sugar because something would need to fill that void. Rather than turning to a different food, my coach helped me come up with a power pose and a power statement to conquer my cravings. She asked me to stand up and explained that physiology plays a big role in how we feel. She described me to a tee. Even though she couldn't see me through the phone, she knew that my shoulders were slumped and my head was down. She asked me what the better version of myself looked like, and I said she was standing tall with her shoulders back and head high with a sparkle in her eye.

My coach then told me to take that stance, plant my feet, place my hand on my hip, and say a power statement together with my power pose. I said, "I can do this," and I felt like a totally different person within seconds. I knew I had to change before I continued to spiral down. I wanted to become the strong Julia who knows the urge is there but does not give in rather than the weak Julia who gives in. I made a choice right then and there to be the stronger version of myself—the one who is empowered and resilient.

For the next two weeks during the detoxification process, I committed to removing all sugars. If the urge hit, I would do my power pose, which became to sit straight, put my hands to my heart, and say my power statement: "Health is my priority. The quality of my life depends on eating quality foods." In order to hold me accountable, we agreed that I would text her three times a day for the first two weeks with positive statements like, "I did it!" or "I got this!" to make the serotonin kick in and make myself more likely to stick to my commitment.

After that session, it felt like a switch went on, and all my cravings for sugar vanished like magic.

Even though I felt powerful, there was a part of me that wondered how long the healthy streak would last. If my past pattern was any indication of the future, it wouldn't last for more than one to two weeks. But during my next session, my coach reassured me that my new identity as powerful Julia could override and replace what I now call the old me. The old me will always be there because my brain will never forget the way I used to behave, but just like that coloring book mentioned earlier, I can color over the old image and eventually build a new picture that looks more like the life I want to live. The image is of a powerful Julia who is smiling her head off because she has so much energy and enthusiasm for life.

Accountability

I thought I could conquer my obsession with sugar on my own. But after five years, I finally came to terms with the fact that I needed more guidance and support.

If you think you have a food addiction, it's important to find someone reliable and committed to helping you. I am really grateful for the support from my Tony Robbins results coach Traci Butz and all the success coaches through the HCI program. Without them, I would not be where I am today. The coaching sessions I had with them were life-changing. Finding a coach is actually easier than people think. Information on finding a match is available in the last chapter of this book.

If finding someone proves to be difficult and journaling is not your thing, you can always count on the universe to support you. You do not have to feel like you are alone. The universe is out there cheering you on.

Text message to the universe: What would you like your power pose and power statement to be?

CHAPTER 10

What Could Happen Because of the Overconsumption of Sugar?

You are free to choose,
but bring awareness to the consequences of your choice.

Picture the garbage can in your kitchen overflowing. There are pieces of food all over your floor, and some of it is rotting and putrid. The more you eat, the more it spreads and rots. Imagine the same thing happening inside your body. Pretty gross, right? The choice to clean things up or leave things as they are is yours. You have the power and ability to make that change.

When we eat excessive amounts of processed food and packaged poison that have no nutritional value, it ferments in the stomach and stops the body from taking in vitamins and nutrients, makes holes in the intestinal lining, and weakens the immune system. But the good news is that the body repairs itself. At some point, though, the body reaches a tipping point, and it cannot heal itself anymore. This is when things take a turn for the worse and people develop poor vision, the onset of diabetes, cancer, or other terminal disease.

Time to Throw Out the Garbage

What can clean things up? Natural fiber from vegetables. Not fiber from powder or laxatives but fresh food—the kind that grows from the ground. But the standard American diet (SAD) does not lend itself to that kind of lifestyle. The acronym SAD says it all. The food pyramid was created by people who were influenced by the food industry, and it desperately needs to be revised. Contrary to popular belief, we do *not* need dairy, meat, pasta, and other damaging foods in our bodies in order to live a well-balanced life. But rather than having someone tell you what to eat or not eat, listen to your body and see how it feels when you eat those things. My body feels lighter without meat, dairy, and flour. The media tells us that we need protein in every meal or carb-filled things in order to make our bodies happy. Is that really true, though?

Many People Are Suffering because of Years and Decades of Not Throwing Out the Trash

Prevention and keeping things clean are the key. If you don't like plain vegetables, add some herbs and spices to them and play around with the flavors or eat them together with something else so you don't taste them. Find your favorite style of cooking vegetables to streamline the cooking process. Do you like them steamed, roasted, sautéed, raw, or juiced?

Try to get a minimum of three servings/cups of vegetables a day, and the best one that has everything you need, including the ability to make you feel full, is kale. There's baby kale, curly kale, and flat kale, and all of it is there for the taking. I like to slice up raw curly kale into small pieces and massage it with some sea salt and sesame oil to soften it up because kale needs tender loving care too. I also like to roast the flat, long-leaf kale in the oven with some coconut oil and eat baby kale with some extra-virgin olive oil infused with basil or rosemary. Sautéing any type of green vegetable with garlic keeps things simple. But don't be afraid to experiment and be creative.

Eventually, your palette will change, and bell peppers will begin to start tasting *super* sweet. Yellow sweet potatoes are very sweet as well. I was pleasantly surprised to see them at Trader Joe's because the only place I saw them was in Korean supermarkets like H Mart, which has all sorts of wonderful, fresh vegetables. Asian markets have a much larger variety of vegetables than American supermarkets, so if there is a big Asian market near you, it is a great place to seek out new foods. Take some time to look around the grocery store, and start with at least one new vegetable to try out. Have some fun!

Word of Caution about Fruits

People grow up thinking that fruit is nature's candy. But how do we eat them with an awareness that there is a lot of sugar in fruit and it can set you off if you are not careful? Why would someone concerned about health not eat fruit? Although fruits contain vitamins and nutrients, sweeter fruits like grapes, pineapples, and pears are high in fructose. Although fructose causes a low rise in blood sugar levels, excessive fructose can lead to the development of metabolic disorders. It all comes down to paying attention to our bodies. Whenever I eat fruit, I start to feel nauseous or my cravings start to kick in. The only fruit I eat is avocados because they are low in fructose even though there are other low fructose fruits like blueberries and other berries.

A word of caution about fresh fruit juices: a glass of apple juice is the equivalent of eating about five apples. The shock to the liver when it gets flooded with all this sugar over and over again could lead to the same type of liver disease as an alcoholic, so please help keep your liver functional by not flooding it with an immense amount of sugar. Store-bought juices are even worse because they have added sugar.

A Lot of Us Know Better, but How Can We Do Better?

The key to preventing autoimmune and other diseases is to keep the immune system strong. Sugar weakens the immune system considerably because the immune system lives primarily in the gut. Genetically modified organism (GMO) products like corn, soy, and wheat can also weaken the system. The overconsumption of antibiotics from factory-farmed animals and fish and prescription medication in addition to the overuse of antibacterial soaps and hand sanitizers are making us sick. It ultimately comes down to building awareness and making better choices in foods and products. Instead of reaching for the quick and easy choice, try to spend some time looking for a better alternative. The extra time spent searching will pay off.

When we feel tired or lack energy, we make compulsive or convenient choices. But avoiding the quick and cheap foods from fast-food burger chains not only helps our bodies, it also helps protect factory-farmed animals, especially cattle. If every family in the United States did not eat meat at least one day out of the week, we could save thousands of animals from being tortured and slaughtered each year and reduce the greenhouse gases that contribute to climate change. We can also preserve natural treasures like the Amazon rainforest from deforestation.

Inflammation

The word *inflammation* comes from the root *inflame* or *set on fire*. The easiest and most visible way to tell that the body is inflamed is through bloating and weight gain. If the body is on fire, something needs to put it out, and one of the best ways is by putting foods in the body that will quell it instead of spreading the flames more. The hardest way to tell that your body is inflamed is through inflammation of the cells. This happens slowly and eventually shows up as autoimmune diseases such celiac disease, Crohn's disease, diabetes, multiple sclerosis, Hashomoto's thyroiditis, lupus, fibromyalgia, rheumatoid arthritis, and cancer. Inflammation is the underlying cause of most chronic illnesses.

Other highly inflammatory foods include dairy, eggs, gluten, peanuts, corn, and soy. Refined carbohydrates in the form of flour, such as wheat flour or rice flour, break down into simple blood sugars during digestion, which raise glucose levels faster than sugar and can also cause inflammation.

Contrary to popular belief, eating fat doesn't make people fat and inflamed. Don't be afraid of eating *healthy* fats from nuts, seeds, avocados, and coconut oil. All of these are needed by the body for proper growth.

Poor Gut Health

Did you know that antacids are the number-one type of medication sold in the United States? Heartburn and indigestion are signs the body sends to signal that it's not well. Antacids are a short-term solution to the problem. The long-term consequences of taking them rather than changing the food you eat could be disastrous.

My husband would pop Tums at least two to three times a week until I told him this little statistic. He finally stopped buying oily muffins and cut down on greasy Chinese food. We used to joke about being hungry within an hour after eating Chinese food and that we would need a second dinner. But now that we look back, it was the sugar that caused the increase in appetite, lack of satiety, and constant search for more food. We called it the Chinese food effect. Now we cook more so we can know what's in our food instead of getting takeout all the time.

Obesity

Excessive weight is a sign of imbalance in the body. When cells store the excess toxins from sugary foods in the form of fat around the organs, it leads to the development of diabetes, heart disease, and joint and bone disease. The source is usually an emotional pattern, so treating the effects of obesity with medication is not going to get to the source of the problem. However, functional medicine doctors can help treat the symptoms because they take a more holistic approach to health. One can search for a practitioner at www.functionalmedicine.org. A health coach can also offer the guidance and encouragement needed. One can search for a coach at www.healthcoachmatch.com

Diabetes

Diabetes has been referred to as a disease of the blood vessels. When the vessels shrink and can no longer get the proper amount of nutrients to the organs, the body starts to shut down. Issues with the production of insulin in the body has become one of the common causes of type 2 diabetes, and some scientists are calling Alzheimer's a form of type 3 diabetes.

According to John Robbins and his book *Diet for a New America*, millions of Americans are suffering from diabetes, and they do not know that their agony could be greatly relieved by different food choices. Because most people eat the standard American diet, within seventeen years of the onset of their illness, most diabetics today suffer a major health catastrophe, such as heart attack, kidney failure, stroke, amputation, or blindness.

The documentary *Carb-Loaded* points out that people who are overweight are not the only ones susceptible to diabetes. Skinny fat people can also develop this disease because of their food and lifestyle choices, so it is crucial for *everyone* to be mindful of food choices.

Dementia and Alzheimer's

If you find yourself constantly being forgetful, it could be your brain telling you that something is wrong. Dementia and Alzheimer's are symptoms connected to the overconsumption of sugar. My grandmother suffered from dementia, which made me determined to do everything possible to prevent the same thing from happening to me. I want to remember who my family members are and continue to enjoy special moments with them in a lucid state.

Changes need to happen now because it takes about fifteen to twenty years for the effects of sugar and processed foods to take full effect. Twenty years from now sounds like a huge amount of time. Come on, seriously. How are the cook__s being eaten now going to affect you twenty years from now? It could, indeed, affect you in the future, and it could also affect you now with high blood pressure or depression.

Depression

Sugar is a depressant. I can't say this enough. It is a stimulant and a depressant, which can be hard to believe, but it's true. Try to detox from sugar for two to four weeks, and see if the dark clouds lift. If that doesn't work, try removing wheat flour, as that is another source of depression. There are people taking antidepressants that cause them to have suicidal thoughts. How is this solving anything? Pills are a short-term solution. Once the pills are gone, the suffering will be back. There is an emotional pattern that needs to be reprogrammed. Perhaps a health coach, other professional, or support group can help break or interrupt that pattern. This could lead to a journey of exploration and discovery that could finally lead to what is missing in your life in order to make it more fulfilling.

There are so many unhappy people who are content with being unhappy.

Do you want to be one of them?

Sugar Addiction Is a Real Thing

Sometimes cravings are really for food and not necessarily something deeper missing in your life. Studies show that sugar is seven to eight times more addictive than cocaine. Dr. Hyman's book *The Blood Sugar Solution* discusses the nature of this type of addiction and how we are a country full of food addicts. The vicious cycles of cravings have led to the consumption of 150 pounds of sugar a year by the average person.

> **Eighty percent of the food in supermarkets have sugar in them, but the 20 percent that don't have sugar are out there for the taking.**

The health of the gut determines the health of the mind, which, in turn, determines the health of the body. If we eat packaged, factory-made food that tears the gut lining, our minds become torn and our bodies are torn apart too. We have the power to make choices, and we can choose to buy foods that will make us whole and well.

Text message to the universe: How can you start making better choices and improve your quality of life?

CHAPTER 11

How Do I Get Toxins Out of My Body so It Can Perform at Its Best?

Breathe in the positive, and breathe out the negative.

According to Ayurveda, toxins in the body come out in various ways, one of which is your tongue. If you see a thick, white film on your tongue upon waking in the morning, it's a positive and negative sign. It's a positive thing because your body is eliminating the toxins, and it's a negative sign because it means you've been putting a lot of toxins into your body.

One of the best ways to get rid of the toxins is by scraping your tongue with either a small stainless-steel spoon or a tongue scraper. All you need to do is gently scrape about five to seven times and remove the film before brushing your teeth. Avoid using a toothbrush to scrape your tongue because the bacteria will end up going back into your mouth.

Detox with Warm Water

According to the *Ayurveda Way*, drinking a small glass of warm water or room-temperature water soon after waking up aids healthy digestion. Drinking warm water before sunrise is said to help reduce hemorrhoids, edema, chronic fever, indigestion, and skin diseases.

One of the easiest and best ways to detoxify is to sip warm water *throughout* the day as well. It allows for the blood to happily circulate in your body versus ice cold water. Imagine sticking your hand into a bucket of ice-cold water. Eventually, your circulation will be affected, and this could cause problems, such as constipation and headaches.

If you are not sure if you are drinking enough water, take the cue from your body. If your urine is clear or slightly yellow, the amount you are drinking is probably enough. Contrary to popular belief, it does *not* have to be eight cups. However, if your urine is a dark yellow color or has a strong odor, your body is telling you it needs more water.

I like to begin and end my day with a cup of warm water. If I feel like I need a little something after dinner, a cup of warm water fills me up and does the job.

Water Infused with Fresh Herbs

If flavor is what you are seeking in your water, try cutting up fresh fruits, mixing them with fresh herbs, and letting them infuse into the water by leaving it in the fridge for at least three hours. Some great combinations include:

- Cucumber and fresh mint leaves
- Watermelon and fresh mint
- Pineapple and rosemary
- Strawberry and basil

Be creative, and create your own combination. Experimentation is what keeps life fun.

Movement

Many people associate movement with getting on a machine and staying there, but it doesn't have to be that way. Get movement in through walking at least thirty minutes a day. It can be in five-, ten-, or fifteen-minute increments for a total of thirty minutes.

If you prefer to do something different, perhaps you could bike, clean the house, dance in your living room, or find a new way to get some movement in. Studies have shown that movements that increase the heart rate lead to an increase in gray and white matter in the brain, and this, in turn, improves memory.

Please don't overdo it when you first start getting more movement in, though. If you do not walk more than ten minutes a day, do not go on a twelve-mile hike for three hours and injure your leg. This is the biggest mistake many people make when they try to become more active. They overdo it, get injured, go out of commission, start making excuses as to why they cannot move, and that's the end of that. If your habit is to sign up for the gym, go every day for a month and then stop going after that. Ask yourself, "Why do I do that?" "What could I do instead?" Perhaps going to the gym one or two times a week for two months might be a better approach. Once you reach new milestones, start to look for different ways to break habits that don't serve you and create new ones that will make you stronger.

Let the Body Rest and Heal During Sleep Mode

Avoid sitting in front of a screen at least one to two hours before going to bed to cut down on the brain stimulation and invest in some blackout liners or curtains to darken your bedroom. Even if all the lights are out, light still filters in through the eyelids and tells the brain that it is not quite time to go to sleep. After I put in blackout curtains, put my alarm clock under my bed, and began to close the door when I went to sleep, I fell asleep much more quickly. I also went into a deeper state of sleep. You know your body is in a deep state of sleep when you dream. I was dreaming like crazy about all sorts of things. I once dreamt that I went back to visit the staff in my old office at Teachers College, Columbia University, and one of my colleagues was upset that the color coding was done incorrectly. When I woke up, I called the office to see how everyone was doing and ask if the color coding was all right. Dreaming prompted me to do something I might otherwise not have done like connecting with people from my past, which was nice.

Your body might work best with seven to eight hours of sleep. Getting too much can be counterproductive. The body heals and restores itself when it is in a state of sleep. Blood sugar balance can also be restored through sleep. Cravings also decrease with more sleep. I can vouch for this statement. I definitely look for less food when I get more shut-eye.

Eat Food That Grows Outside

Where can things that nourish us and give us energy come from? Most people cringe and say they can't eat vegetables all day, but it doesn't have to be that way (unless you would like to, which your body would thank you for). The body needs the fiber and the nutrients from vegetables if it is going to scrub the intestines and clean out the digestive tract.

How to Know if Your Bowel Movements Are Up to Speed

According to Ayurveda, the waste inside your body should be removed on a daily basis through regular bowel movements. The stool should be soft and log-shaped and not have an odor. Hard stools or runny diarrhea are signs that the gut is not well. Millions of Americans suffer from constipation because of the lack of fiber in their diets. Who wants to eat broccoli or kale when there's a burger that has lettuce and tomato? The small amount of lettuce and tomato are not going to cut it, unfortunately.

I joke around with my kids and ask them if they have done their daily doodie to make sure that they are getting enough vegetables. They think it's weird that I ask them if they have pooped on a daily basis, but that's the only way I know that they are okay. If people in your family are not having one to two bowel movements on a daily basis, it is a sign that waste inside the body is not being removed properly. Before it becomes a red flag in the form of hemorrhoids, it's important to find ways to add more natural fiber from the *v* word, the *v* word being vegetables.

There are a lot of creative ways to stick some extra veggies into dishes like pureeing some zucchini and mixing it in an organic pasta sauce that doesn't have sugar or simply roasting some cauliflower by tossing it in coconut oil, sprinkling it with a little salt, and putting it into the toaster oven for thirty minutes until the tops become a little brown. I couldn't believe it when my son ate the entire cauliflower the first time I made it.

I learned that if I put vegetables on the table and don't say anything, they are more likely to eat them than if I beg them to eat. If people don't reach for it at first even with a little prodding, they will eventually get used to seeing it on the table and try it. They say that it takes twelve tries before kids will try a new food. I wish I had known this when my kids were really young because I usually gave up after three or four tries. But if you let them know that vegetables have to be part of every dinner and/or lunch, they will grow up with the same mindset, and you will be helping them in the long run.

If you are a parent who doesn't like eating vegetables, is it because of the way you grew up? Studies show that this would indeed be the case because how you eat in childhood is how you end up eating in adulthood. It's critical that the importance of eating fresh food becomes ingrained in the brain at an early age to avoid pain and suffering later. I know that I have a tendency to repeat some concepts over and over, but it is done intentionally because studies also show that in order for the brain to remember something for a longer period of time, it needs to be exposed to it at least three times.

Dry Brushing

If you do suffer from constipation, there are some natural ways to get things moving, such as dry brushing. This technique has many other added benefits, including relief from joint pain and improved blood circulation.

Dry brushing involves using a dry body brush (the type for showers) and using short, quick strokes toward your heart starting on one side of the body. I find that brushes feel a little rough, so I use a small kitchen cloth instead of a brush. I start on my left hand and swipe each finger with the cloth and then flip my hand and swipe the other side of my hand. I then swipe my wrist, up my arm, and toward my head. Then I go to my left foot and swipe up my leg toward my heart. After I am done with one side, I do the same thing on the other side of the body and then the belly area, shoulders, and the rest of the torso. This technique is easy and can be done in less than three minutes. There are many videos on YouTube that explain how dry brushing works that can be helpful.

Oil Pulling

Oil pulling entails swishing around a spoon of either coconut oil or sesame oil in your mouth for ten to twenty minutes in the morning when your stomach is empty. I used to think the concept of this was sort of strange, but I have found that it does help with a lot of different things, including removing the morning bacteria inside the mouth, strengthening the gums, and reducing signs of plaque. After swishing the oil around, I spit the coconut oil out into a paper towel or the trash can. Spitting it out into the sink is *not* recommended because once the oil hardens, it could clog the pipes. After spitting it out, I rinse my mouth with water at least three times, and that's it.

A Note about Coconut Products

I am a huge fan of using coconut oil in many different ways. It has so many natural antibacterial properties. I use it as a hand sanitizer, lip balm, and in lieu of lotion for my hands when they get really dry. I also use it as a substitute for cough medicine when my son is sick. I either give him half a teaspoon of it or put a spoon of the oil in a cup of warm water with a little bit of freshly squeezed lemon juice.

Coconut oil has also been known to lower cholesterol, aid with digestion, and aid in liver health. That's why I cook with it all the time. When I want to add a rich coconut flavor to the food, I use the unrefined kind. On days when I would prefer not to taste the coconut, I use the refined kind. The better choice is the unrefined, though because it has gone through less processing. It is high in saturated fat and can be cooked at high temperatures, which makes it great for baking as well. However, if you have never eaten coconut oil before, start with one tablespoon a day because there are side effects to the overconsumption of the oil such as dizziness, stomach upset, and fatigue.

Coconut water is great for quenching thirst because it has natural electrolytes. It's a much better choice over energy drinks filled with sugar and salt, which end up depleting electrolytes. Coconut water is also a natural laxative, so please be careful with the overconsumption of this drink.

Coconut milk is divine with a sprinkling of cardamom and turmeric. Both of these can be found in the spice section of some supermarkets. A tiny amount of cardamom goes a long way. I find it to be a great alternative to sugar, but it has a very unique flavor that takes a little getting used to. My taste buds have changed a lot, and things that are typically not that sweet can taste very sweet. You will also find that your taste buds change after about one to two weeks.

Experimentation

If you haven't noticed any real differences in your body after the six- to eight-week mark, I would recommend doing an elimination diet or experiment. Begin by removing one particular type of food for two to four weeks and then reintroducing it slowly and noting any differences or just not consuming them anymore. I would recommend eliminating dairy products first, which would include yogurt, milk, cheese, etc.

Other foods to eliminate completely for two to four weeks after your first experiment could be sugar, wheat flour, corn, and/or soy. Only eliminate one type of food at a time for a specified period of time and become aware of how your body feels. This is a great way to detox the body.

Ultimately, patience is the key. The word *patience* itself can trigger impatience, but we must be peaceful with ourselves and our bodies as we start to learn more about the interconnectedness between the gut, mind, and heart. The cultivation of health, well-being, and inner peace progresses over time and doesn't really end.

Mental Detox

A mental detox can have tremendous benefits that can help further the whole-body detox. When my coaches helped me to detox from the negative feelings, regrets, and resentments I harbored, it felt really great to let it all go and forgive—forgive myself, forgive others, and just release all the negative energy and thoughts that had been lingering for years. As a result of the coaching sessions, I decided to grow my heart and seek out kindness.

Text message to the universe: How do you plan to get toxins out of your body?

CHAPTER 12

How Can I Continue to Enjoy Food Without the Sweet Factor?

At first, they'll ask why you're doing it.
Later, they'll ask how you did it!

I was walking down the supermarket aisle one day and saw a couple of people looking at the ingredient list on an item. If more and more people did this, there would be fewer and fewer ill people, which would be such a wonderful thing. I love shopping at organic stores because there are so many wonderful foods that don't have sugar, but I am seeing an upward trend in the number of products with sugar or sweeteners, so I hope it doesn't keep happening.

Here are some tips on how to enjoy food:

Focus on what you can eat

Instead of focusing on what you cannot eat, focus on what's in front of you and what you can eat. If you start to get into the habit of enjoying the vegetable soup instead of feeling like you are missing out on the chowder that everyone else is having, your body will thank you because you won't feel heavy afterward and wake up lethargic.

Chew

The longer you chew something, the more satisfying it will be. It will also last you longer, so you don't feel hungry as quickly. Chewing food until it becomes a pulp instead of simply swallowing it and letting it slide down is also better for digestive health. Digestion begins in the mouth when the enzymes start to break down the food, so if you don't feel well after eating, chewing thoroughly might help you feel better!

Eat *mindfully*

What does eating mindfully entail? It means *savoring* the food by using your five senses and chewing mindfully. The book *Mindless Eating: Why We Eat More than We Think* by Brian Wansink is a fun read with a lot of great ways to eat less mindlessly. The more mindful you are of what you are eating, the more satisfied you will feel, so it will make you less likely to look for additional food. Avoid eating out of a bag or box while sitting in front of a screen. I purchased small containers that are equal to about one serving size and make my kids pour the food into them to avoid overeating.

How long do you spend eating lunch? The first time I timed myself, it took me seven minutes. Nowadays, so many people eat on the go or at their desks that spending more than ten minutes eating feels like a luxury. People are sick and stressed because they are woofing things down faster than someone can sing a song.

Next time you eat lunch, time yourself. Seriously. See how long it takes you to eat from start to finish. If you spend less than five minutes, try to add on at least five minutes by taking some extra time to chew. If you can build up to twenty minutes of chewing, eating mindfully, and relaxing while you eat, your body will start to turn the wheels. If you are extra mindful, you will start to notice the benefits.

Finding *Sweetness* in Life

Sweetness can be found in things other than food. The next time someone does something nice for you, take a moment to appreciate the kind gesture or words. Find something to savor as often as possible, and before you know it, you'll find that food isn't the only way to find sweetness. I used to try and savor the moment by looking at an old photo for more than a few seconds.

Studies show that doing nice things for others makes us feel uplifted. Holding the door for someone can make us feel happy.

Try to put things in a new perspective. A sweet treat after lunch could be fresh air outside or a walk around the block with the sun shining down. Find things that make you smile, and hold onto that feeling for as long as possible.

Text message to the universe: How can you find sweetness in things other than food?

CHAPTER 13

How Can I Continue to Rewire My Brain?

When you feel like quitting, remind yourself why you started.

Habits that meet strong needs are particularly likely to come back, according to the book *Making Habits, Breaking Habits* by Jeremy Dean. So if you find that you are having a really hard time breaking the habit you chose, there is something very deeply ingrained that you are trying to hold onto and don't want to let go. What could it be? Is it because it's part of your identity?

The ridges in your brain will always stay where they are even though new ones form, so if you find yourself going back to your old ways, just know that this is okay. Don't give yourself a hard time about this, and more importantly, don't give up on yourself because this happened once or more. It took me two years to break my habit of needing a little something after dinner, and I regressed quite a few times—a lot of times if I am going to be completely honest. But now that I finally broke the habit, it feels great to feel a new sense of freedom.

Rather than focusing on suppressing your old habit, try to work with it. See it as a friend who keeps coming over. Ask it why it keeps coming by nicely and approach it with curiosity rather than contempt or anger. Eventually, it will stay a shorter time because it will feel bored that it can't get under your skin anymore.

If you have ever been a teacher, it's like that student who acts up because they want attention. They will get it whatever way they can. But once positive reinforcement sets in and is repeated, the student will turn around, and the worst kid in the class could become the model student. It happened in my class when I used to teach at a middle school in New York. This particular boy was the shortest, loudest, and most disruptive kid in my social studies class, but I pegged him as a leader. The other students did what he did, so I told him that I thought he could be a great leader. This completely threw him off, but slowly he became less disruptive, and so did the other students.

I have learned that I create my own misery. I could dislike everything that the student did and wish I was sick every day so I wouldn't have to go to school and teach, but I could create my own happy place as well. Rather than blaming others for my woes, I chose to do something that would be more empowering for him and for me.

Here are some other ways to pave the way toward a more empowering lifestyle:

- Get into the habit of asking yourself, "Will this help me or hurt me?" Eventually, the brain will learn to stay away from things that hurt you.

- Congratulate yourself on little things, such as saying, "I'll pass for now," to someone who offers you something sugary. That is a huge accomplishment!

- Live life with a grateful heart, and be thankful for the body you do have instead of living from a place of lack. People who feel that they are lucky are much more resilient.

- Trade in judgment and criticism for curiosity and compassion. (I am my own best friend instead of my worst enemy. This finally happened during a success coach call when my coach told me to put my hand to my heart and ask myself how I could love myself more.)

- Make it a team effort. Having other family members, friends, or colleagues on a path toward wellness will make things much easier. Surround yourself with like-minded people and find places where you can meet them by going to www. meetup.com.

- Accept yourself and your situation, and then look for ways to evolve and grow.

- Love yourself by putting your hands on top of your heart and making a promise to take care of your body, accept it, and love it.

- Acknowledge that your brain wants to keep you safe and will resist change.

- Anticipate and prepare for resistance by the inner voice. Talk to the negative inner voice in a compassionate way and ask what it needs.

- Going back to old ways will be part of the journey, and it is not a setback. Accept that it happened, try to learn from it, and carry on.

- Send positive vibes to the universe that you will feel amazing one day, and that one day can become multiple days, weeks, months, and years.

- Make self-care a priority for at least five minutes a day or at least thirty minutes a week. Your spouse and kids will see the payoff with a calmer you.

- Grow your mind. Read self-development books or write your own book.

- Listen to motivational speakers like Tony Robbins and Mel Robbins.

- View progress and changes as positive forces saying hello to your new, better self.

- Don't let negative people halt your journey. A significant other may not want you to lose weight or feel better because they want to maintain status quo. A change in you might mean changes for them, and some people fear change like the plague. Assure them that there will be some really awesome things happening for everyone.

= Brain Activation Mode = BAM

The above list is pretty long, but is there anything that stood out that you would be willing to try to reprogram your brain?

If not, what could be something else you could try?

Think possibilities.

Text message to the universe: What is one thing you can *commit* to in order to rewire your brain?

CHAPTER 14

How Should I Handle Food Boredom and Deprivation?

If nothing changes, nothing changes.
—Courtney Stevens

I never thought of myself as an emotional eater. Then I learned that eating out of pure boredom also fell under the emotional eating category. I would eat when I felt bored and had nothing to do, and when I experienced something I call *food boredom*, I would reach for processed food because I felt bored with the foods I was eating. I didn't really eat the same food all the time except maybe nuts and seeds because it's my go to food when I feel a little hungry before or after a meal. But when I got bored of eating any vegetable even though it was a different one every day, I searched for something else in the form of something sweet or salty.

Dealing with Food Boredom

After numerous sabotaging sagas with food boredom, I realized my consumption of nuts and seeds happened just about every day and not just a few days a week. I have started a new rule that doesn't allow me to eat the same food more than two days in a row because I don't want to fall back into the habit loop and feel bored again.

So now that I don't eat the same food two days in a row, things have been nipped into bud. If I had pumpkin seeds two days in a row for breakfast, then I'll eat some almonds the third day or some mixed nuts. And I try to eat different colors of vegetables on different days.

Dealing with Deprivation

After all the yo-yo dieting to try and shed the last ten pounds, I found myself overeating out of frustration and anger. There had to be a reason why I couldn't lose the weight no matter how hard I tried, so I just said, "What the hell. I already ate a bite, so I might as well finish the rest of it." I was using the what-the-hell effect to justify why I couldn't lose weight. I didn't like this new habit and who I was *being* when I did this and who I was *becoming*, so I tried yet another program that claimed it wasn't a weight-loss program even though it was designed to help women lose weight. I learned what I could, but I went back to my old ways eventually.

One day, my sister mentioned a health coaching program that she was interested in, and I thought, *Hmm … Why not do a health coaching program and focus on my own self-care? When I am ready, I will be able to help others.* After I enrolled in the Health Coach Institute (HCI), I learned that stressing about losing weight causes the body to hold onto the weight. *Darn it*, I thought. *So I have been having a hard time losing the weight because I was stressed about getting the weight off?* Yes. It's true. I saw a quote that said the best diet is the one you don't know you are on. So I decided to put away the scale, throw away the packaged food in the house, buy tea, and just be. Before I knew it, my pants felt looser, and I felt happier.

But the *biggest* takeaway from the health coaching program was trading in judgment for curiosity. Asking questions such as, "What is missing in my life?" and "What needs to be nourished?" helped me to move forward in the healing process. I have searched and searched for the answers, and every day, week, and month it was something different. Sometimes I didn't have answers, but I learned that it's okay not to have the answers. I just decided that I was tired of hiding and wanted more from life.

= Brain Activation Mode = BAM

When you eat sweet tasting foods, what are you trying to escape from? Hide from?

What's stopping you from finding inner peace?

Then ask yourself, "What can I do about it?"

Think possibilities.

The old me used to be impulsive and eat things whenever she wanted; the newer, more powerful Julia is someone who is resourceful and capable and who makes health a priority and doesn't make excuses. Instead of being frustrated because I couldn't go back in time and have my prebaby body back, I decided to focus on improving my present situation. Once I made that decision, it was as if the universe heard me and started sending a lot of different resources my way such as self-development books, stories of inspiring women, mind and body programs, and a health/life coach.

Keystone Habits Are the Key

When I got into the habit of using positive self-talk, my life started to turn around and become more fulfilling. If we turn something into a keystone habit, it sets off a chain of multiple positive habits and outcomes. For example, by talking to myself compassionately, I started to believe that changing my career would allow me to grow and reach new heights. The doubts and fear were replaced by positive thoughts that made me believe I could write a book and break free from all my sugar habits. The creation of keystone habits can be a crucial part of a personal development journey.

In Charles Duhigg's book *The Power of Habit*, he discusses how a keystone habit such as habitually exercising even just once a week can start changing other unrelated patterns in a person's life, often unknowingly. Typically, people who exercise start eating better and become more productive at work. They feel less stressed and show more patience to colleagues and family. Exercise is a keystone habit that triggers widespread change.

At the core of why those keystone habits were so effective is the concept of a small win, according to Duhigg. Once a small win is accomplished, we are driven to want another win. Small wins fuel transformative changes that convince people that bigger achievements are within reach.

= Brain Activation Mode = BAM

Is there a keystone habit such as getting more sleep, eliminating negative self-talk, replacing the perfectionist mindset, eliminating excuse making, saving more money, packing lunch, preparing meals in advance, or a different one that you would like to commit to?

Think possibilities.

Look for More Possibilities

Everyone is born worthy. Worthiness is not something that has to be earned. Everyone has it and begins on the same, level field.

It's people's *mindsets* that takes them to where they end up. Some people see many choices and possibilities in life. They are the people who end up thinking of themselves as worthy. Others end up feeling trapped with no choices and no possibilities. These are the people who feel they have to prove or earn their worth in order to be accepted and offered choices. They wait for others to change their lives for them instead of feeling like they can do it themselves. But all of this is just an illusion. It's a story that took hold and hasn't left. It's time to change your story if the latter is the case.

There is no need to hide your true self anymore. Take off your masks and your hats and accept yourself and your situation. Awareness and acceptance are the keys to making progress.

Text message to the universe: How would you like your life story to change?

CHAPTER 15

How Can I Improve My Quality of Life?

Old ways won't open new doors.

Transformation can happen within minutes, but the transformational journey takes months, years… a lifetime. If you have ever watched the movie *The Matrix*, one of the premises is that people get bored when their lives are perfect, so they need struggles and conflicts. Sometimes we have to wonder why we have to struggle, but I believe that all of our lives' experiences lead us to a certain point where we can cumulatively use those experiences and transform them into something more.

If I hadn't struggled for all these years, I wouldn't have come upon the 5 Second Rule or the concept of tapping and many other wonderful, game-changing strategies.

The 5 Second Rule

The 5 Second Rule helps remove the mental habit of hesitating. The book *The 5 Second Rule* by Mel Robbins provides many different examples of how millions of people around the world utilized this rule to stop hesitating and move forward with their goals. (The brain hesitates to protect us and keep us safe.)

When Mel Robbins was about to lose her house and everything she had, she suddenly decided to count down five, four, three, two, one, and launched off her bed one morning like a rocket. Her life has never been the same since that one moment. If you have a goal and hesitation stops you, just count down from five and go. Move your body physically, and do something that would help achieve that goal. After I heard this, I tried it the next day, and I launched myself out of bed so fast that I didn't even know what happened. I used the rule to conquer my sugar habits. I have also used the rule to calm myself down in order to be a better wife and mom. When I feel the irritation rising in my voice, I count down from five and respond to an argumentative question raised by one of my kids v-e-r-y s-l-o-w-l-y. The first time I did this, my son asked me why I was talking so slowly, and I told him that I was trying to stay c-a-l-m, and then we both laughed.

Self-Development Books

The key to meeting a long-term goal is to focus on progress rather than the outcome. With each passing day, we become someone different. We might feel like the same person because we all have our habits and lifestyles, but if we want to keep growing and transforming, we have to be open-minded and look for ways to acquire new knowledge. I have never read so many self-development books in a one-year span. These types of books are also called self-help books. I stayed away from them at first because I didn't want to think of myself as someone who needed help.

The first book I read was *The Power of Habit: Why We Do What We Do in Life and Business* by Charles Duhigg. I enjoyed reading this book because it explains how the brain works when it comes to habits. I felt so much better knowing that it wasn't just me and my brain that couldn't figure things out.

I wasn't a big fan of audiobooks because I couldn't keep up with who was who, as I was multitasking and not fully focusing. But then I decided to listen to *You Are a Badass: How to Stop Doubting Your Greatness and Start Living an Awesome Life* by Jen Sincero, and I realized that self-development books were much easier to follow than novels. This book changed my life and inspired me to write a book of my own. I want people to experience what it's like to live an awesome life. I believe that *everyone* is capable of being amazing in their own way and not just a select few.

Empowering Questions

If we get into the habit of asking ourselves high-quality questions that empower us, it can change our mindset dramatically. Instead of asking disempowering questions like, "What's wrong with me?" try asking, "What can I do to make my life even more fulfilling?" This question implies that you already find your life fulfilling, but you would love to get even more out of life. High-quality questions lead to a high-quality life, according to Tony Robbins.

Whenever something unexpected happens or I get stuck in traffic, I have started getting into the habit of asking myself, "What could be great about this?" I then pinpoint at least one thing, and it brings peace and calm to the situation rather than irritation. I once went to an event that was scheduled for a certain time and got an email less than a day before stating that the start time was being moved up by thirty minutes. I arrived early just to learn that the original time was indeed the correct time. So I went outside and asked myself what could be great about this. I decided to go for a walk, do my mind is like the sky meditation as I walked, and explore the area. I really enjoyed having the extra time to do this and take in the extra sunshine.

See Life as a Gift and Live in the Present

If you see life as a gift, you will enjoy the present. This is what the book *The Gift of Our Compulsions: A Revolutionary Approach to Self-Acceptance and Healing* by Mary O'Malley has taught me. By replacing *mindlessness* with *mindfulness* through the five senses and taking the time to smell the peppermint tea and taste it while holding the warm cup and looking at the white clouds in the blue sky while hearing the birds chirping, we can be more present. The more we do this even though our mind wanders and the more we accept our situation, the more fulfilling our lives will feel.

Move Away from Perfection and Accept Imperfection

The book *How to Be an Imperfectionist* by Guise states that perfectionism creates feelings of guilt, anxiety, inferiority, and irritability. On the other hand, imperfectionism creates feelings of satisfaction, happiness, and calm. The big determinant on how you choose to live depends on what you care about.

The mindset of imperfectionists:

- Care less about results.
- Care less about problems—just take them as they come. Care more about making progress, being resourceful, and finding solutions.
- Care less about what other people think. Care more about who you want to be and what you want to do.
- Care less about doing it right. Care more about doing it at all.
- Care less about failure. If something didn't work, try it in a different way.

In general, imperfectionism is about caring less about certain things and focusing more on how to move forward with your identity and your life. Once I moved away from the perfectionist mindset, it was as if all the burdens that were on my shoulders started to lighten, and my daily activities didn't feel like arduous chores. Instead of stressing out about completing everything on my to-do list perfectly, I decided that just getting it done was more important. For example, instead of spending thirty minutes crafting a perfect email, I decided to limit myself to five minutes and keep it succinct. I love living life as an imperfectionist.

Tapping

Tapping is more formally known as Emotional Freedom Technique (EFT). This technique has been used with veterans for post-traumatic stress disorder (PTSD) and many other types of conditions. Tapping helps lower stress by decreasing cortisol levels by 20 to 50 percent. It can also decrease food cravings and essentially improve your relationship with food.

Tapping involves using your index and middle fingers to gently tap eight meridian points in your body to clear up blockages and access your body's healing power. The eight meridian points are: 1) the tip of the eyebrow closest to the nose, 2) side of the eye, 3) under the eye (above the cheekbone), 4) under the nose, 5) chin (below the lip), 6) one inch below the collarbone, 7) underneath the armpit, and 8) the very top of the head. Tapping these eight points about five to seven times very gently is almost like doing acupuncture without needles.

I usually start with the right side of my body while saying how I feel and then saying a positive affirmation, such as, "My body can heal on its own." Then I tap the left side, and then I use both hands and tap both sides at the same time. I use this rotation for about five to fifteen minutes. You can do all the tapping on one side instead of rotating, but I think that changing sides taps into more parts of the body. But that's just my preference. I tap when I am not feeling well or when I can't fall asleep, and I always feel better afterward because I *believe* in the healing power of tapping.

Watching videos on how to tap online and following along can also be helpful in order to get a better sense of how tapping works.

Text message to the universe: How do you plan to improve your quality of life?

3
PART

HOW TO MAKE NEW HABITS STICK

CHAPTER 16

How Can I Become More Resilient?

What if … everything you are going through is
preparing you for what you asked for?

There are numerous ways to generate brain power in order to achieve optimal self-regulation. Visualization and mental rehearsals are powerful tools that can help you stay on your ride. I started to believe in the power of these mind tools after watching the third episode of the *Transcendence: Live Life Beyond the Ordinary* documentary series through Food Matters TV (FMTV). During the cycling portion of a triathlon, Joe Dispenza shattered his spine after being hit by a vehicle. His doctors told him that he would never walk again, but he refused surgery and pushed out thoughts of being in a body cast for a year and being handicapped for the rest of his life. He opted for mind and body connection techniques and reconstructed his spine with his mind. Miraculously, he was back on his feet in ten weeks. Miracles sometimes happen on a whim, but miracles like this require special forces that have to come from within the individual.

Visualization and mental rehearsals are really
powerful tools if you believe in them.

The Power of Habit by Duhigg references mental rehearsals that Michael Phelps utilized to prepare for the Olympics. His coach told him to turn on the video and mentally rehearse what the perfect lap would feel like, as well as rehearse laps that could take the wrong turn. In one of the competitions, Phelps had to swim blindly because his goggles filled up with water. What could have been a disaster ended up earning him a gold medal and a new world record.

Visualization

Visualization ignites the power of possibility. If you visualize yourself doing something you've been wanting to achieve, your mind will automatically seek and attract things that will help you achieve your vision. Visualization usually entails creating a positive image in your mind and using the five senses to make that image as real as possible. I would picture myself doing a book talk at Barnes & Noble and holding my newly published book in my hand. There were many times when I wanted to put writing a book on an indefinite hold, but I wouldn't let myself do it because something inside of me told me that I could make that image real.

Mental Rehearsal

A mental rehearsal is a little different from a visualization exercise in that there is more action. It is usually used by athletes to practice a certain skill like throwing a basketball from the three-point mark (without physically doing it), but it can be used in many different contexts and take different forms. You can choose to see yourself as a third party watching from the outside in, or you can choose to be the person acting out the part.

While I was obtaining by health coach certificate, my wonderful success coach Tracy Hjorth did a mental rehearsal with me when I was feeling confused and lost. She had me find a quiet spot where I would not be disturbed and could be honest with myself. She then had me close my eyes, take a couple of deep breaths, and picture a golden light shining above my head sprinkling me with warmth.

About five feet in front of me, I was asked to picture a future version of myself one year from that day. I saw a version of myself with a sparkle in her eye, skin that was glowing from happiness and enthusiasm, and a genuine smile because she was thrilled that she made it. I have never seen myself so happy, and it made me want to cry.

My coach then asked me to slip my fingers into her fingers and my toes into her toes and feel her heartbeat. Once I became my future self, she coached me by asking what the future Julia was looking at, and I told her that she was looking at a Julia who was crying on the couch. The future me asked why I was crying, and I told her that even though I had made a lot of progress in finding peace with myself and food, I felt like I was starting to regress and was starting to feel disempowered, lost, and stuck.

My coach asked the present me what I would like to ask the future me, and after a heartfelt conversation, the future me told me to trust her and that she would help me get to where I wanted to be. I believed her.

We ended by giving each other a hug.

I did this at least once a week on my own before falling asleep and in the morning upon waking for the next month. When I felt lost or confused, I did a mental rehearsal with either the future, present, or past version of myself. I have found that this is a really powerful way to build self-compassion.

I have read so many books that tell people to be their own best friend, but I have never really been able to do this. But merging with my future self and knowing that she won't give up on me no matter what happens is really empowering.

If you have never done a mental rehearsal before, following the steps I took in the example I just gave can be helpful. But if you can find a coach or someone you trust to walk you through a mental rehearsal, it can be even more powerful. Ultimately, the answers are inside of you, and you are the only one who can draw them out. Talking to yourself in a compassionate way instead of a condescending way brings forth feelings of reassurance and resilience that are resolute.

It was kind of strange talking with the future me, and even though I ardently told her that I wanted to give up, she refused to let me. The genuine resolve and belief that she had in me that I could do what I set out to do wouldn't let the present me give up. I think I was partly able to do this because I didn't see the future version of myself as a stranger who wasn't real. I knew in my heart that she could be real, and I would be able to feel what she was feeling. When I talked with the past version of myself, I realized that instead of trying to find the old version who felt great at one point in time long ago, it would be wiser to let go of the past and step up to the next phase of life.

Resilience and Compassion

Building resilience and compassion through mental images can be very empowering. The brain depends on symbols and images to plot out its course. If it constantly sees you in a certain way, it will generate the power to actualize that image.

Text message to the universe: What would you tell your future self if she or he was standing in front of you?

CHAPTER 17

What Can I Do to Keep Sugar Out?

What I am aware of, I can change.

Whenever my husband does the grocery shopping, he comes back with junk food 40 percent of the time. Thankfully, he has dramatically reduced the amount he buys, but the bottom line is that he still buys it. I used to think he was the end of me and saw him as a mean enabler. How could someone who claims that he loves me be trying to end my life?! He knows what sugar does to me and how if I see it, I want to eat it. When I told my results coach about this, she compared bringing sugar home to bringing alcohol home to an alcoholic. If the urge resurfaced, my brain would go off like fireworks, and eating sugar would be like having a relapse. She suggested that I have an honest conversation with him and find ways to compromise.

I finally decided to take responsibility for my own actions and stop playing the blame game with my husband because it wasn't helping in anyway. So I tried to put the healthier stuff at eye level and hide the processed stuff toward the top, bottom, or back of the shelves. This worked for a while. Then I decided to put the junk in a totally different cabinet. This has helped a lot. Other people in the house are just not ready to be where I am in my journey, and it's not fair to expect them to be, so looking for solutions and compromises instead of griping about the problems is my new thing, and it has really helped.

When I go to the supermarket, I avoid the middle aisles because that is where the dangerous foods call out people's names. If something sugary calls out to me, I turn myself around and keep telling myself that I don't need it. I have found that if I look at it for too long or touch it, I become very tempted to buy it, so now it's a no-touchy situation.

When I pass on buying something, I smile and actually feel proud of myself. Celebrating the little victories is really the key to making new habits stick.

If you used to buy sugary stuff impulsively and now you think about it before putting it in the cart or don't put it in the cart at all, that's huge!

It's really important to find something to celebrate *every day*. Not doing this will feel like there is no purpose to your actions and that you are depriving yourself. Feelings of deprivation will eventually be replaced with feelings of empowerment because you are taking control of your health.

Become an Educated Consumer

Nutritional labels can be tricky to decipher, so it's best to keep things simple.

1. Avoid items that have the different names for sugar and artificial sweeteners on the ingredient list.
2. Avoid items that have words you can't pronounce

= Brain Activation Mode = BAM

If you are the gatekeeper in the family or the person who does the grocery shopping, what is something you could do differently next time you are at the market?

If you are not the gatekeeper, how can you make sure there are fresh foods and healthy choices at home?

Think possibilities.

Just Follow the Recipe

The concept of family mealtime is disappearing. The convenience and abundance of frozen dinners and takeout has replaced home-cooked meals. But we can change that. Start by cooking one simple meal at home just once a week. Most supermarkets have recipes on their websites, so something could be chosen from there. They will even deliver the groceries, so you don't have to stress about going out and buying the ingredients.

I have always thought of myself as a crummy cook. This has been ingrained as part of my identity, but I found ways to change that belief.

I have finally committed to following recipes step-by-step. I would constantly deviate from the recipe and leave things out or add things because I thought my way would be healthier, but the kids refused to eat what I made. Now that I stick to the recipe, people actually eat it. There are websites with recipes that have four ingredients or fewer, which can make things much easier. I have also found that linking a pleasant activity with cooking, such as humming or listening to music, makes the time in the kitchen more enjoyable.

Cooking and Eating Together as a Family

The best way to empower children is to teach them how to be self-sufficient. My family divides responsibilities, and we take turns preparing the meals and cleaning the dishes. Asking kids to pitch in, even if it's just to peel a cucumber, can give them the power to feel like they can do something for the greater good. If they peel the cucumber in a funny way, just thank them; otherwise, getting them into the kitchen again will be very difficult.

When I was growing up, my mother and grandmother took care of all the cooking. But I realized that not knowing the ins and outs of cooking made me want to stay out of the kitchen as an adult. Feeling incompetent doesn't feel good, but learning a new skill does feel good.

When my family sits to eat and talk about our day, my kids know to eat the number of vegetables that corresponds to their age. So when they were five years old, they had to eat five pieces of vegetable that were on the table. This worked really well, and now they eat vegetables for dinner every night because it is a habit for them. I will be thrilled if they are doing this when they are forty years-old.

Stress at Work

Stress at work is a big reason why people seek out sweet or salty stuff. It sends the brain on a reward-seeking mission, which usually sends us on a never-ending habit loop. We need to feel a little relief and want to avoid feeling disappointed, so a trip to the coffee machine or vending machine gives us that. What if vending machines or coffee machines didn't exist? What might you do instead if you need a break?

Instead of walking to the vending machine, how about asking colleagues if they want to grab a cup of water and take a quick break or go for a quick walk around the block? Remember that it's important to replace one habit with something else. Simply stopping the 3:30 break to the vending machine will work a few times, but then chances are that you will go back to that habit instead of breaking free from it. If you tell your brain that there are alternatives that are better and you enforce this with feelings of accomplishment, the brain will feel more at ease and say, "Okay, it looks like you got this."

According to *The Blood Sugar Solution* book, how we handle stress dictates the length and the quality of our lives. Chronic stress causes the brain to shrink and the belly to grow. Cortisol shrinks the memory center and activates a biological response that results in hunger.

Acknowledging the stress and the craving and using breathing techniques or other mindfulness techniques to put the body into relaxation mode can calm the brain faster than resisting the urge. Relaxation mode reduces cortisol levels and allows us to lessen cravings.

What to Do When You Are Out

American culture puts a lot of emphasis on food as the medium that brings people together. So what should we do when we are faced with a ton of food that we don't want to eat in order to join the crowd and feel like we belong?

It begins with a change in mindset. Rather than focusing on the need to belong by eating food others are eating, focus on *connecting* with the people who are there and having conversations with them. When we talk with each other, food actually gets in the way because it can be messy or it might get stuck in our teeth. In reality, no one is paying attention to what you are eating or how much of it you are eating. If it is on their radar because they made the dish, thank them and smile and say how delicious it smells. This approach might mean more to them than seeing you eat it.

Restaurants

If you are going to a restaurant, try to look at the menu online beforehand. This will allow you to make the better choice in advance when you are not under time pressure or when you are hungry. If nothing seems appealing, eat something before you get there and then order a couple of side dishes. I usually order two to three side dishes as my meal because that's where the steamed broccoli or better choices can usually be found. I love it when I see the option of ordering side dishes as a meal on the menu itself.

Skip the sugary drink, appetizer, and dessert because those are all unnecessary. When I am out with friends and everyone is ordering drinks except for me, I just say that I will start with water. When dessert time comes, I just get tea. Portion control is so out of control that the main dish could feed two or three people, so there is no need to feel like you should order a drink, appetizer, and dessert just because everyone else is ordering them. Who knows—maybe next time, the other people will skip those too.

Below are some guidelines on how you can make the better choice if you are faced with a decision between two dishes. Choose the item that has:

- Less sauce (a lot of sauces have added sugars)
- More vegetables
- No dairy*

*The protein casein and whey in dairy creates a whole host of other problems in addition to the lactose.

Text message to the universe: What can you do to keep sugar out?

CHAPTER 18

How Can I Develop More Brain Power and Self-Regulation?

Don't wish it was easier. Make yourself stronger.

When we try to forbid ourselves or try to rid our minds of something, it boomerangs back. One solution could include developing enough brain power and self-regulation techniques to acknowledge the urges and temptations. Please note that I used the word *acknowledge*, not *fight* or *push away* because having a fight with yourself inside your brain is not going to end peacefully. The word *fight* in and of itself implies violence and winners and losers. We are not looking to see who will win at the end of the ordeal. We are simply seeking peace.

Peace can be found in many peaceful ways. Breathing deeply, meditating/staying still, sleeping, and moving allow the mind to develop the brain power. These forms of energy management can help reduce the stress response and the need to focus on immediate forms of gratification.

Stress Relief Switch

Stress can drain willpower very quickly. The fight-or-flight response is a form of energy management that makes us focus on the immediate things. The brain is set up for survival, not happiness. This is why habit disorders such as excessive eating or drinking can lead to many types of mental issues like anxiety and depression or physical issues like gastrointestinal disorders and back pain. So what can we do? We can build in mindfulness practices to help us not only survive but to thrive. We really need to take a step back and give ourselves a break and turn on the stress *relief* switch. Reducing stress will make you crave less and make you feel more in control of your life in general.

Building Mindfulness Practices

What does being mindful entail? It entails having awareness of the present moment and accepting it in a nonjudgmental way. How can we do this? The good news is that there are a variety of ways, and it can be done in one minute or one night.

Breathing Techniques

Did you know that there are a lot of different ways to breathe? People who are stressed breathe in a shallow way from the chest. People who are more relaxed take deeper breaths from the diaphragm. Take a moment to notice how you breathe. When you take a deep breath in, does your belly go in or out?

When we were babies, we were born breathing the correct way: When you breathe in, your stomach should push out so you can open up your diaphragm. But then as we get older, we stop breathing that way and don't take in the oxygen and let out the carbon dioxide to keep the body in balance.

There is a technique called the 5-5-7 breath where you count 5 seconds while you breathe in, hold for 5 seconds, and then exhale for 7 seconds. There is another one called the 5-5 breath where you count up to 5 while breathing in and then count down from 5 while breathing out. There are a million variations. The key is to take deep breaths and open up your body.

Stress is the number-one cause of illness in the United States. It causes all sorts of major imbalances. My friend's husband has been to every single type of doctor and has had every single type of test to find the source of his migraines, digestive problems, insomnia, and a million other symptoms, but the doctors can't find anything wrong. Stress is most likely the thing lurking in all his cells. It has to act out because it is tired of not getting the break it needs.

Power breathing doesn't have to happen in a yoga class. It can happen when you are walking down the hall or driving in your car. Research shows that deep breathing makes you more resilient to stress and increases the willpower reserve. All of this can happen in just *one* minute.

One powerful way to boost self-regulation is by slowing the breath to four to six deep inhales and exhales per minute.

I have gotten into the habit of taking deep breaths for at least one minute upon waking and one minute before falling asleep. I have found that waking up and doing this sets the tone for the day and puts closure at the end of the day.

Breathe in Possibilities (BIP)

At different points during the day, I also try to breathe in positive energy and breathe out the negative energy. The more we practice being in the moment, the easier it becomes to control our impulses. I have started calling this practice BIP, which stands for Breathe in Possibilities. Please take a moment to BIP now: Take a deep breath in and in your head say, "Breathe in possibilities." And then exhale slowly. If we remind ourselves that we have choices, it puts our minds more at ease.

Be a Seeker of Stillness

Many people find the concept of meditation intimating. I used to find the word itself intimidating. The word made me feel like I had to be a certain kind of person in order to be able to meditate, but that is not the case at all. Perhaps calling it something else will be less intimidating, like stay-still time.

A meditation practice or stay-still time includes: 1) Staying still (this works self-control/impulse control), and 2) Focusing on the breath (feeling the sensation of your breath going in and out of your nose or saying the words *inhale* and *exhale* to bring your mind back when it wanders; bringing the wandering mind back is a form of self-control as well).

If doing these at the same time is unnerving for a long period of time like it used to be for me, practice doing these steps for one minute and build from there. Closing your eyes or glancing down and either sitting upright or lying down can help calm the mind and body. Breathing in through the nose is recommended and breathing out through either the mouth or nose is up to the seeker of stillness.

Be sure to schedule it either in the morning or at night or when you can find one to five minutes to stay still, such as before you eat lunch. Starting in an easy, doable way is the key to sticking with it.

Benefits of Staying Still

I have learned that the goal of staying still is not to clear the mind. It's to be present in the moment and cultivate a positive state of mind.

Staying still is a way to practice a greater degree of awareness: It increases attention, self-awareness, and self-control by increasing the blood flow to the prefrontal cortex and building up that brain power. Practicing a form of mindfulness can put a stop to the habit loops that can take us on detours.

After months of quasi staying still, I attended a retreat called "Change Your Mind, Change Your Life" at the Kadampa Meditation Center in Texas led by a warm-hearted Buddhist monk. I always thought that the goal of meditating was to focus with the mind, but after attending the retreat, I learned that the ultimate goal is to grow the heart.

I also learned that meditation improves the quality of our minds, the quality of our lives, and the quality of our daily experiences. It can also improve the quality of our relationships because if we can be at peace with ourselves, we can be at peace with others. I left the retreat with a heart full of love and compassion for others; it was truly an enlightening experience.

The secret to total fulfillment is to accept our true selves.

In meditation, we connect with our true selves, and eventually this allows us to strengthen the connections we have with others.

Building Mindfulness in Schools

If schools sent children to meditation sessions instead of detention in order to improve self-regulation skills or offer mindfulness as part of the curriculum or as an after-school program, there is a very good chance we would have more productive students and happier teachers. Although mindfulness is not meant to be a behavior-modification technique, it can lead to a greater sense of calm and teaches students to respond to triggers thoughtfully rather than react impulsively. By zooming out of a situation and pressing the pause button, mindfulness allows us to see more choices. Perhaps building mindfulness is the secret to higher rates of graduation and teacher retention. Anyone and everyone can benefit from mindfulness practices, and more and more studies are showing this.

After experiencing the benefits of meditating, I wondered how I could share and teach others the transformative nature of something so simple. I got my sign from the universe when I got an email from Mindful Schools stating that a certificate was available as a mindful educator. I knew right then and there that this was how I could help people in a meaningful way, so I signed up that day. It was as if the universe prepared me to share this powerful practice by allowing me to experience being a teacher when I first got out of college and then working with educators at the higher education level. I truly believe that mindfulness sessions should be included in every new teacher orientation to help teachers manage the feelings of overwhelm in a way that makes them feel empowered.

Nearly 50 percent of new teachers leave the profession within their first five years, which calculates to millions of dollars in losses by school districts, but more importantly, thousands of hours of quality instructional time are lost due to teacher burnout and absenteeism. When I facilitate mindfulness sessions, my intention is to share practices that calm the mind through awareness of the present in nonjudgmental ways.

Restorative Sleep

Sleep deprivation decreases the ability to self-regulate and interferes with how the brain and body manage energy. According to *The Willpower Instinct*, a single good night of sleep can replenish willpower, and a single night of bad sleep can do the opposite—one night.

The Willpower Instinct book recommends *relaxing* even for just a few minutes by taking in deep breaths or sipping warm water to restore the willpower reserve. In this case, relaxing means tuning out to external stimuli rather than sitting in front of the screen or drinking an alcoholic beverage.

Journaling

I wish I could buy all the inspirational journals that are in Barnes & Noble and Staples. I love how mindfulness journals are becoming more available because we could really use them to figure out how to live life to the fullest. My current journal has the words "DREAM big, SPARKLE more, SHINE bright" on the cover in gold lettering and a soft beige cover, which I love holding in my hand. It is filled with my attempts to work through challenges and find solutions, as well as stick figures of me going up and down jagged lines as I search for the ultimate path in life to make it epic. Keeping a journal has helped me see problems as opportunities to learn; this shift in perspective has been instrumental in helping my mind think from different angles.

According to *The Blood Sugar Solution*, keeping track of your feelings and habits in a journal creates a system of feedback and accountability that can be healing and helps change behavior. I would recommend getting a journal that you like holding in your hands and start writing!

Send Positive Vibes to the Universe

Whenever I send positive vibes to the universe, it always comes through. When I was looking for a new house, I made myself believe that I would find a house with everything I wanted, and I did! If you truly, in the deepest part of your soul, believe that whatever you want will manifest itself, the universe will make it happen. Staying positive in this way has helped build resilience because I see setbacks as opportunities to develop more patience. After we put an offer on the first house we liked, we didn't get it because the owners had already verbally promised it to another family. Instead of getting upset or sad, I just had a feeling that this had happened for a reason. The next day I walked into the *perfect* house. I just knew it was the one! I kept thinking and saying, "I am going to send positive vibes to the universe for the perfect house," with all the conviction I could muster, and the universe delivered. When you feel like things are not in your favor, just know the universe is always on your side.

Live Life with Gratitude and Appreciation

In a competitive world where we constantly strive for more and are made to feel like what we have is not enough, it can be difficult to be grateful for what we do have and appreciate the people and things around us. Many of us look for material things to bring us joy, but in order to really experience happiness, we need to cultivate it inside of us.

The Mindfulness Awareness Research Center at the University of California Los Angeles (UCLA) has been coming out with research that an attitude of gratitude changes the molecular structure of the brain, keeps gray matter functioning, and makes us healthier and happier, which, in turn, affects our central nervous system and makes us feel more peaceful and less reactive. If we choose to live from a place of gratitude instead of lack, we can be more present and appreciate life more.

Be Sweet

When we get out of our own worlds and into someone else's, it connects us to our common humanity, according to Dr. Mark Hyman in his book *The Blood Sugar Solution*. Science shows that altruism activates the same reward pathways in the brain as sugar but without all the negative side effects. Finding a way to pitch in and satisfy the human need to be of service also provides a deep sense of happiness.

If you volunteer for different activities but want to do something more consistently and contribute in a more purposeful way, consider sharing your knowledge and skills by giving free talks at libraries, churches, or other community organizations about something you love to do or can help people do better like how to start and grow a business or how to be calmer around kids. If there is something you have been interested in learning more about, teach yourself something new and share what you learned with others. Whether three people show up or fifty, focus on impact and being of service rather than numbers. If speaking in front of a large group of people is not quite your thing, limit the number of people who can register; start small, and focus on presence and what you can offer instead of what people will think of you. I love it when people come up to me after a workshop because lifting people up is what life is all about.

If teaching others in public is a little daunting at the moment, start by gathering one or more friends, family, or kids and teaching them cooking tricks or sharing breathing techniques.

There are a lot of creative ways to be of service and share a message, so allow your voice to be heard and your actions to be seen and *be* sweet, so the world can be a sweet place to live.

Be Curious Instead of Judgmental

The brain likes to play games. Sometimes it comes across in mean ways through negative self-talk and a judgmental tone. But if you can play the brain game in a way that is advantageous to you by being curious instead of judgmental, you can outwit your own brain. What a thought! So instead of, "I will always be fat, and I will never be good enough," how about replacing judgmental statements with curiosity by asking questions. For example: Why do I need this ice cr__m at night while I watch television? What do I really want? Is the ice cr__m a substitute for companionship? Is eating it a way to fill the emptiness because I feel like nothing I do matters and that no one really cares what I do or don't do? What is missing in my life that requires me to seek solace and escape through food?

Once you have pondered the questions, what are some empowering alternatives to your current habit? Instead of watching television and eating ice cr__m, what could you do that would make you feel better? If you are craving companionship, maybe you could look for a Meetup or start your own! After I moved halfway across the country and did not know anyone in the new area, I joined different Meetup groups. I love how there is always somewhere I can go to be with like-minded people. The way people support and encourage each other at the different activities and events is heartwarming, and the people who I have befriended have enriched my life.

If you are craving more knowledge and growth, enroll in an online class or consider becoming a health coach. I never saw myself as the coach type, but I've learned the power of transformation through these programs. Making a personal investment in myself made me feel like I matter, and I want to help others feel like they matter. Find something that will help grow your mind and skills. If you like cooking or want to learn more about cooking, look for bloggers or cooking classes or offer your services as a private or personal chef. I have found that looking through Facebook feeds is a great way to get new ideas and check out new possibilities.

Move Around to Make Your Brain Bigger

A pedometer is a great gadget that can help make you walk at least ten thousand steps per day. If ten thousand seems daunting, start at five hundred or any number that you see as doable. When you pass that number, smile and say, "I did it!" Once again, doing this is what will make you keep going. Don't compare yourself to others and how much they walk. Just focus on you and the building of your ride, and every time you pass your old number, be proud of your accomplishment.

If there's a day when you don't feel like moving, just count down—five, four, three, two, one—in your head and then say *go* and physically move or do something. The 5 Second Rule can work here too if you need that little extra push to meet your movement goal.

The benefits of movement are immediate, and some call it a wonder drug. Fifteen minutes of getting your heart rate up decreases cravings, is an antidepressant, and makes your brain bigger. Start by committing to walking around the block once a week until you are ready or happy to add more time. Shorter bursts that make your heart pound have a more powerful effect than longer periods of time, so turn on your favorite song and go around the block.

Movement also helps with blood sugar stability and boosts serotonin levels, which helps prevent depression. Moving your body makes you breathe deeper, which oxygenates your body and mind. You've got nothing to lose and a lot to gain by walking. Do circles around your living room, or put on your sandals, sneakers, or whatever you've got and get some fresh air into your lungs.

If you like working out in groups but worry too much about what others will think of you, I found the perfect quote for you by James Purpura: "You can stop worrying about what other people think of you. They are too busy worrying about what you think of them."

Focus on your health and your body. If the others want to be judgmental, so be it. Once everyone leaves the gym, their thoughts go out the door too. But how about greeting people near you with a smile and a hello after you walk into the class? You will be surprised by how different the atmosphere becomes with this simple shift. Instead of a judgment zone, it becomes a let's-do-this-together-because-we-made-it-here zone.

When I go to the gym, I am the one in the back corner modifying everything. Jumping jacks are done moving one leg at a time. I never jump. That's just how I roll. I don't use any weights, and I don't use a step for step classes because I have been in four car accidents. (None of them were my fault. The most recent one was with a guy on his cell phone. He crashed into me when I came to a stop because of traffic.) But it's not about making excuses. I could use that as my excuse, but I know my body and what makes it feel better and what makes it feel worse. Not moving and not stretching makes me feel tight and achy, so I will opt to move it moderately.

What kind of movement is right for you? What type of movement do you want to do today? What kind of movement did you like to do as a kid? Are there other people you could do activities with? What is something you have always wanted to try?

Create your own movement menu, and keep things fun!

- Walk around the block and look at the sky before getting your mail.

- Try a dance fusion class at a gym and move to the music instead of worrying about keeping up with the moves. (If you can't keep up, just walk in place. This is totally okay!)
- Play the song "Let It Go" from the movie *Frozen* and pretend you are Elsa.

= Brain Activation Mode = BAM

Which one or more of the choices above (deep breathing, staying still, sleeping, journaling, sending positive vibes to the universe, living with gratitude, being sweet, being curious, or moving) could you try this week?

If you already incorporate mindfulness practices in your life, how could you develop them further or be more consistent about them?

Think possibilities.

= Beyond BAM =

How could using mindfulness practices help your mood? Your life?

How would having more brain power and better self-regulation help you?

Text message to the universe: What's something you can commit to this week that would make you feel calmer and more at peace?

CHAPTER 19

How Can I Continue to Evolve and Shine?

Appreciate and model kindness.

According to Dr. Sean Stephenson, there are two ways to feel good. You can find gratification based on the principle of finding pleasure now and pain later, or you can find *fulfillment* based on the principle of putting in effort now and pleasure later.

> The only person who can make you feel powerful is *you*.
> The only person who can make you feel miserable is *you*.
> You have more power than you think.
> What you do with that power is totally up to *you*.

If you can't see the big picture, then you are too zoomed in. In order to see the bigger picture, you must zoom out. Rather than wondering why this is happening *to me*, reframing the situation and seeing it as happening *for me* can make all the difference. It would be great if struggle didn't have to be painful, but the wisdom gained from being able to overcome the struggle can perhaps lead to a passion project that will allow others to learn from your experiences. Sharing your insights and inspiring others can be a gift you can share with the world.

Moving from Habit Change to Lifestyle Change

If you would like to move from habit-change mode to lifestyle-change mode, give your brain a heads-up that there will be some changes and more positive things happening soon. Just tell the brain that you are going to do some cleaning. If you are the type of person who likes cleaning, even better! You are going to clean out the pantry, fridge, and freezer and take away the sugary temptations. If your keystone habit was or will be to buy things less impulsively, your home should naturally fill up with healthier items.

Before embarking on your journey toward freedom from harmful habits, it is really important to prepare yourself mentally. After many frustrating attempts at breaking free from sugar, I have learned that mental preparation is just as important or even more important than the physical preparation.

It's time to be resourceful and find ways to live the life you truly desire.

What I Learned

After my five-year journey trying to get away from the pain sugar causes my mind and my body, I've learned to link sugar with *severe* pain and a low quality of life, so I have vowed not to go back to my sugar habits again. I think I could have shortened the journey by focusing on shifting one habit first, then setting up a keystone habit, and then committing to some integral lifestyle changes instead of trying to quit sugar all at once. But my journey has brought me to where I am today. True transformation occurs when we look inward, build self-compassion, and move toward a more positive mindset. When we look to our hearts for kindness, compassion, and gratitude, life feels like a gift filled with possibilities.

I recently came to the realization that trying to be a higher version of myself and trying to upgrade to Julia 3.0 can have some repercussions. I learned that when we strive to be a better version of ourselves, we are rejecting who we are, which increases feelings of inadequacy and not being enough and brings forth more judgment. There's a fine line between striving to be better and *choosing* to live a life of increased well-being by practicing kindness. I choose kindness.

Embrace a Positive and Resilient Mindset

Transformation begins in the mind. Study after study shows that a positive mindset can lead to positive outcomes. Rather than fighting the negative inner voice, listening to it with compassion and calming it by letting it know you are safe can help reframe things in a way that will lift you up rather than throw you down. Being honest with ourselves is hard. It puts us in a vulnerable place. But surrendering does not equal defeat. Surrendering to what your body and the universe are trying to tell you can lead to a greater sense of resilience and empowerment.

= Brain Activation Mode = BAM

In order to feel fulfilled in life, there are three questions to ask:

1. What can I do to grow and stretch? Could it be by learning more about mindfulness, visualization, or a new language?
2. What types of human interactions do I value? Is it laughing with friends, holding someone's hand, or smiling at someone and receiving a smile back?
3. What can I do that will allow me to feel the human interactions I value?

Think possibilities.

Acknowledge that you do make a difference. The type of difference you make will be up to you. There will never be another you. Use your heart, story, and experiences to make an impact. This can be in the form of a conversation with someone about the impact of food on the body, or perhaps it could be on a larger scale through workshops or events. Devote yourself to service in a way that calls out to you.

Investing in a Health Coach or Life Coach

If you are not sure how to feel more fulfilled, perhaps a health coach or life coach could bring out parts of you that you didn't know existed. I would recommend someone from the Health Coach Institute (HCI), so they can support you at the transformational level because they have been trained to be masters of habit change. You can find a coach via Health Coach Match at www.healthcoachmatch. com. You can search for someone near you or anywhere in the world and connect with them via computer or phone. Many of the health coaches hold dual certifications as life coaches.

There are also coaches through the Tony Robbins Results Coaching Program at www.tonyrobbins.com/coaching who can catapult you to the next level of your life. There is only one you who can do what you do. All you need is a mind that can look for possibilities.

When you are searching for a coach, look for someone who can point out your blind spots. What habits and patterns are you not aware of that are hurting your quality of life? Look for a coach who will take on a holistic approach to wellness and will guide you in finding empowering ways to cope rather than someone who will take an advice-giving approach, give you a list of things to try, and tell you to see how it goes. They might provide temporary solutions, but that's all it will be: temporary.

A majority of coaches offer free initial conversations, so you can find a coach who matches your needs. The cost of a coach can be quite high depending on who you choose, but the investment you make in yourself will pay off for the rest of your life. Not just your life—the people around you will also benefit from the positivity you embrace. As a result of having amazing coaches, I have turned my thinking around and have learned to live with more compassion for others. I have even found ways to appreciate my husband more than I did before. Once the inner work begins and takes hold, the benefits to the outer world and people around us start to show up in wonderful ways.

We All Have a Little Light Inside of Us

All of us, not just some of us, have a little light inside of us that has either dimmed or is waiting to come out and shine. I hope this book has created a little spark within you that will ignite dormant energy that can take you on a lifelong journey toward a powerful you. Your body and your mind are the greatest instruments you will ever own. You have the rest of your life to transform them in ways you never thought possible. Keep learning, keep growing, and keep building up.

One day, I hope you will share your message with others and lift them up.

Think possibilities. Think positivity.

Text message to the universe: What would you like the universe to know?

APPENDIX

Appendix A: Sugar Habit Tracker

The first step in breaking free from the sugar habit is to **become aware** of when you consume sugar.

Write down the time of day and food or drink that has sugar or artificial sweeteners over the course of 3 to 6 days. Once this is done, circle any patterns you notice.

Note: If printing this sheet from my website is not possible, simply draw 3 columns on a sheet of paper.

Day 1	Day 2	Day 3

Sugar Habit Tracker

Please continue to write down the time of day and food or drink that has sugar or artificial sweeteners. Once this is done, check to see if you have a sugar habit by circling any repetitive patterns you notice.

Day 4	Day 5	Day 6

Appendix B: Body Scan Log

When you wake up and open your eyes, before you even get out of bed, take 1-2 minutes to do a body scan. Starting at the top of the head, check in to see how you feel. Does your head feel heavy? Do you feel pressure behind the eyes? Does your nose feel stuffy? Is your mouth dry? Check in with the rest of your body and continue with your neck, shoulders, back, arms, belly, legs, and feet.

Day of the week:

Body scan results:

Energy level upon waking: High — Okay — Low — Deplorable

Day of the week:

Body scan results:

Energy level upon waking: High — Okay — Low — Deplorable

Day of the week:

Body scan results:

Energy level upon waking: High — Okay — Low — Deplorable

BIBLIOGRAPHY

Ajmera, Ananta. *The Ayurveda Way: 108 Practices from the World's Oldest Healing System for Better Sleep, Less Stress, Optimal Digestion, and More.* North Adams: Storey Publishing, 2017.

Dean, Jeremy. *Making Habits, Breaking Habits: Why We Do Things, Why We Don't, and How to Make Any Change Stick.* Boston: Da Capo Press, 2013.

Duhigg, Charles. *The Power of Habit: Why We Do What We Do in Life and Business.* New York: Random House, 2012.

Guise, Stephen. *How to Be an Imperfectionist: The New Way to Self-Acceptance, Fearless Living, and Freedom from Perfectionism.* Columbus: Selective Entertainment, LLC, 2015.

Hyman, Mark. *The Blood Sugar Solution: The UltraHealthy Program for Losing Weight, Preventing Disease, and Feeling Great Now!* New York: Little, Brown and Company, 2012.

McGonigal, Kelly. *The Willpower Instinct: How Self-Control Works, Why It Matters, and What You Can Do to Get More of It.* New York: Penguin Group, 2012.

O'Malley, Mary. *The Gift of Our Compulsions: A Revolutionary Approach to Self-Acceptance and Healing.* Novato: New World Library, 2004.

Robbins, Anthony. *Awaken the Giant Within*. New York: Simon & Schuster, 1991.

Robbins, John. *Diet for a New America: How Your Food Choices Affect Your Health, Happiness and the Future of Life on Earth*. Novato: New World Library, 1987.

Robbins, Mel. *The 5 Second Rule: Transform Your Life, Work, and Confidence with Everyday Courage*. US: Savio Republic, 2017.

Rubin, Gretchen. *Better Than Before: What I Learned about Making and Breaking Habits—To Sleep More, Quit Sugar, Procrastinate Less, and Generally Build a Happier Life*. New York: Broadway Books, 2015.

Wansink, Brian. *Mindless Eating: Why We Eat More than We Think*. New York: Bantam, 2006.

RECOMMENDED READINGS

Books about Habits and Mindset

The 5 Second Rule: Transform Your Life, Work, and Confidence with Everyday Courage by Mel Robbins

Better Than Before: What I Learned about Making and Breaking Habits—To Sleep More, Quit Sugar, Procrastinate Less, and Generally Build a Happier Life by Gretchen Rubin

The Gift of Our Compulsions: A Revolutionary Approach to Self-Acceptance and Healing by Mary O'Malley

How to Be an Imperfectionist: The New Way to Self-Acceptance, Fearless Living, and Freedom from Perfectionism by Stephen Guise

Making Habits, Breaking Habits: Why We Do Things, Why We Don't, and How to Make Any Change Stick by Jeremy Dean

Mindless Eating: Why We Eat More than We Think by Brian Wansink

Mindset: The New Psychology of Success by Carol Dweck

The Power of Habit: Why We Do What We Do in Life and Business by Charles Duhigg

The Willpower Instinct: How Self-Control Works, Why It Matters, and What You Can Do to Get More of It by Kelly McGonigal

Books That Will Lead to Better Health

The Ayurveda Way: 108 Practices from the World's Oldest Healing System for Better Sleep, Less Stress, Optimal Digestion, and More by Ananta Ajmera

The Blood Sugar Solution 10-Day Detox Diet: Activate Your Body's Natural Ability to Burn Fat and Lose Weight Fast by Mark Hyman

The Blood Sugar Solution: The UltraHealthy Program for Losing Weight, Preventing Disease, and Feeling Great Now! by Mark Hyman

Diet for a New America: How Your Food Choices Affect Your Health, Happiness and the Future of Life on Earth by John Robbins

I Quit Sugar by Sarah Wilson

Wheat Belly Journal: Track Your Path Back to Health by William Davis

Books That Will Lift Your Spirits

Awaken the Giant Within by Anthony Robbins

The Universe Has Your Back by Gabrielle Bernstein

You Are a Badass: How to Stop Doubting Your Greatness and Start Living an Awesome Life by Jen Sincero

You Can Heal Your Life by Louise Hay

Printed in the United States
By Bookmasters